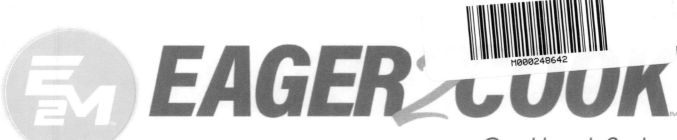

EAGER2COOK™

Cookbook Series

Healthy Recipes
for Healthy Living

**Seafood
& Salads**

SPARK Publications
Charlotte, North Carolina

Eager 2 Cook™: Healthy Recipes for Healthy Living
Seafood & Salads
E2M Chef Connect LLC

Eager 2 Cook™ series by Golden Spoon Holdings, LLC

The E2M program provides suggestions on eating a whole food diet that has successfully helped tens of thousands of members achieve their weight loss goals. Before you start this or any program, consult with your physician to clear if this program is a fit for you, your body, and your health, taking into account allergies, pregnancy, or any other physical condition. The content in this book is intended to be generally informative and not provide medical or nutritional advice, and has not been evaluated by physicians, nutritionists, or the Food and Drug Administration (FDA). The E2M program makes no healing claims and does not guarantee any health or weight loss successes. Resulting meals depend on preparation and ingredients used, and the E2M program or cookbooks make no warranty regarding the outcome of your use of these recipes.

Designed, produced, and published by
SPARK Publications
SPARKpublications.com
Charlotte, North Carolina

Written by: Chef Jennie Casselman and Chef Andres Chaparro

Photography by: Shane Amoroson

Printed in the United States of America

Paperback, January 2023, ISBN: 978-1-953555-44-1
eBook, February 2023, ISBN: 978-1-953555-45-8

Library of Congress Control Number: 2022923118

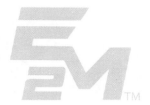

Dedication

I dedicate this book to all the people
who believed in me. With positive support
anything is possible, and the people in my
life who support my wild ideas give me the
fuel to chase my dreams each day. I would
not be successful without you. Thank you.

Jeff Witherspoon

Table of
Contents

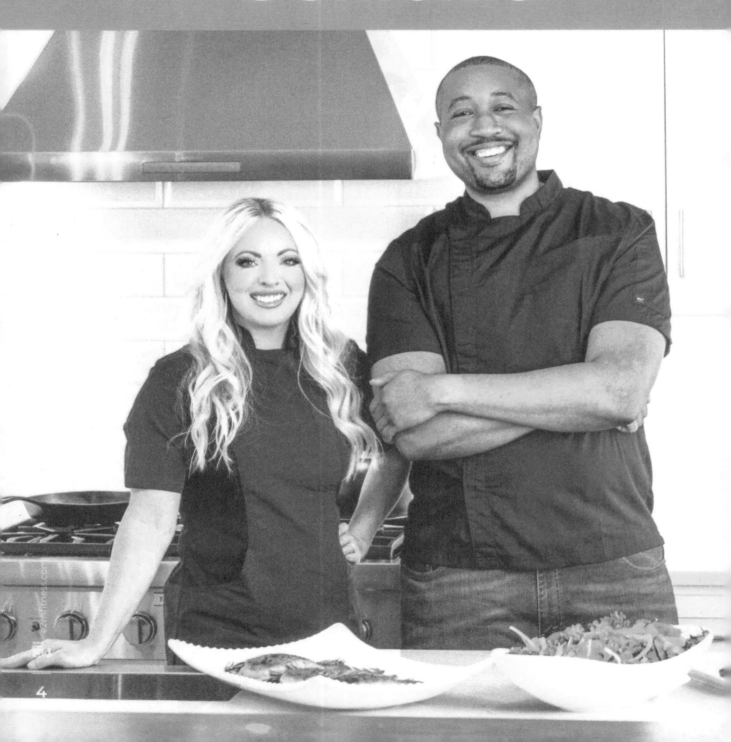

e2mfitness.com

Salads 83

Dressings

Spice Blends

Introduction to
E2M™ Fitness

What is the E2M™ Program?

It is a virtual, eight-week, rapid body transformation program for adults, which consists of workouts, meal plans, cooking classes, mental fitness, and personal coaching. Workouts are designed for all levels and *abilities and can be done at home or a gym. Meal plans* vary from week to week and are free of supplements, using only whole, nutrient-dense foods. Our meal plans can accommodate any dietary restrictions, including postpartum recovery and vegan. Each member gains access to certified fitness coaches and thousands of other program members who make up our fitness community. Our Fit Family is made up of people across the world from various backgrounds and age demographics, but what we have in common is one goal: to encourage each other to reach our personal best lifestyle and fitness goals. And after the first eight weeks, the program is available for free to maintain progress.

This isn't about getting "skinny" or "beach ready"; it's about building a healthier lifestyle, living longer, and getting the most out of the body you've been given. This is a lifestyle of health and wellness, and we have the tools to support you in every step of your journey. Whether you want to lose a few pounds, tone up and get stronger, or learn how to sustain a healthier lifestyle with your family, we'd love to help you.

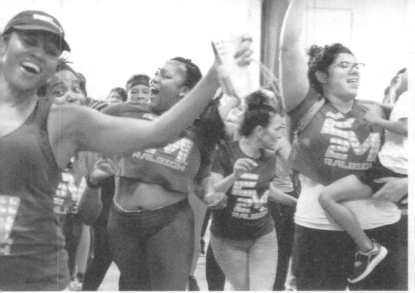

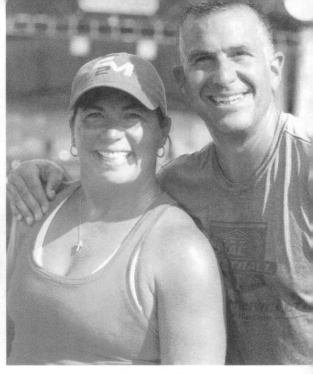

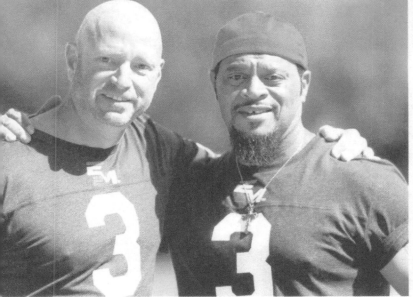

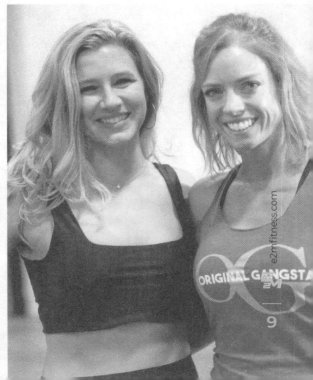

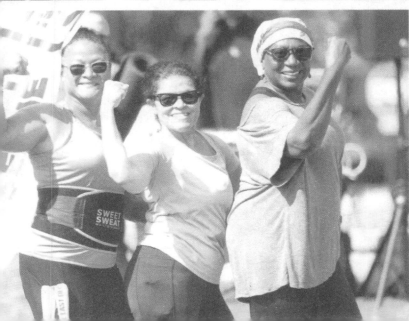

e2mfitness.com

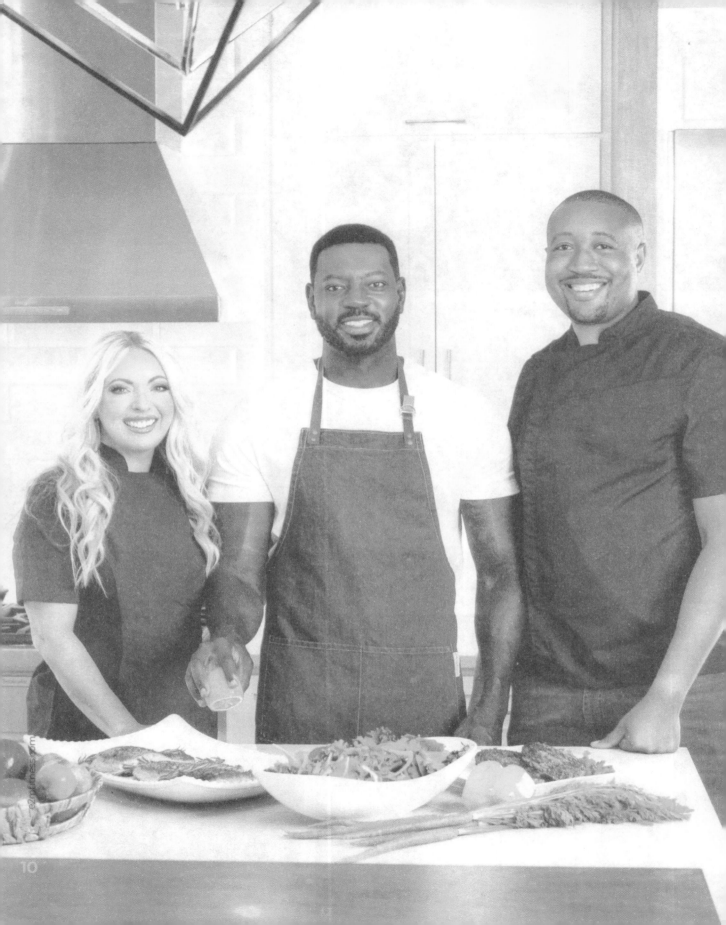

Note to
Members

To my amazing E2M fitness family, we did it!

This cookbook would not be possible without you. It is my sincere hope that this cookbook becomes another tool you can use to maintain your health for years to come. The chefs put lots of time into this and I am excited to see even better results now that you can be a little more creative and still stay on plan. Cooking can be time consuming, but learning to love the process of preparing healthy meals to fuel your body can make cooking your new hobby.

These cookbooks are for us but not only for us, so feel free to recommend the cookbooks to your family and friends because they need to eat healthy too, and they just might end up joining the E2M family. As you improve your health, your life will also improve. JUST KEEP TRYING. Finally, thank you to our amazing chefs Jennie and Andres! They wanted to share some E2M community favorite recipes, and some new ones, in a usable format to make life easier and being healthy more enjoyable. I hope you love what we put together.

Jeff Witherspoon

"It is my goal to help as many people as possible, and I can't wait to help you improve your health, improve your life! I look forward to the chance to be your guide on your journey to your optimal health and fitness."

— JEFF WITHERSPOON

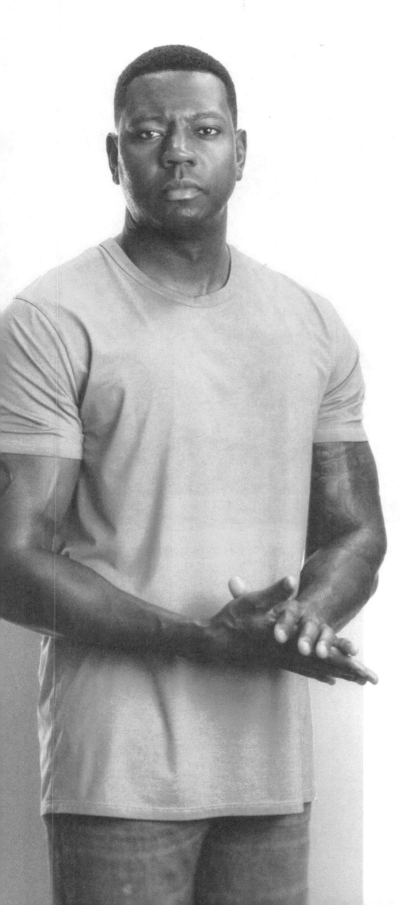

Jeff Witherspoon

Owner, Founder

Jeff Witherspoon's fitness journey began when he was a young athlete at The Citadel in Charleston, South Carolina. Jeff received a full-ride scholarship and worked without ceasing to quickly become a champion track-and-field athlete. He found great joy in bringing home numerous wins for the Bulldogs.

Upon graduation, Jeff began a successful career in the army as a field artillery officer; he has served our country in several overseas tours. While on a deployment, he found fitness as a way to cope with the stresses of combat. He enjoyed not only the way that working out made his body look but also the way that focusing on his health made him feel. Jeff found that "fitness became a place of release and therapy." Fitness enabled him to manage high levels of stress in the military and to handle more stress in a positive way.

Later in his career, Jeff became a certified hand-to-hand combat instructor for the army. This certification and practice introduced him to another form of fitness and discipline that he also enjoyed. This new level of discipline would eventually permeate all areas of his life.

As Jeff began to encourage fellow soldiers and friends to work out and eat healthy, he recognized his passion to help others. Fitness and nutrition became tools he used to help lead other soldiers with PTSD in coping with day-to-day stressors and to assist them in improving their overall health and wellness. This sparked his desire to become a certified personal trainer.

Jeff's passion and business grew as he began to see how his knowledge and motivation were helping others transform their lives. Providing accurate and factual advice to improve others' fitness levels is his main goal. Through all his experiences, he strategically created what is now E2M Fitness, a worldwide fitness program changing lives one day at a time.

e2mfitness.com

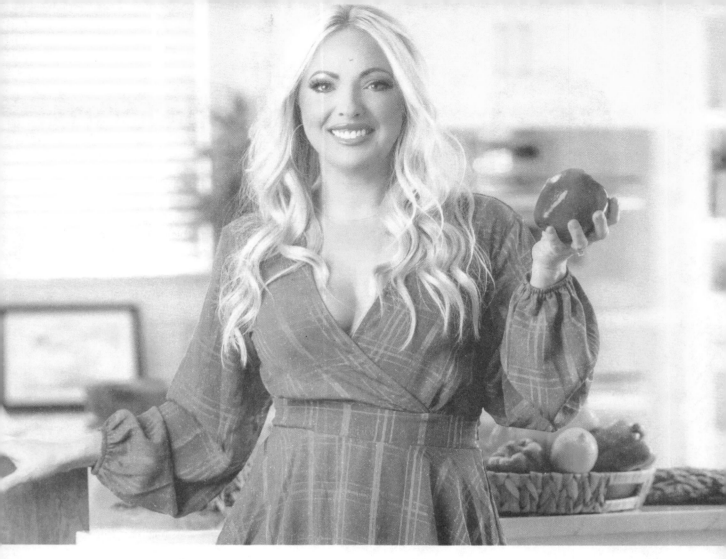

Jennie Casselman

Chef & NASM Certified Nutrition Coach

Growing up in a large southern family, Jennie always enjoyed being in the kitchen with her mom. "I was raised in a family who honored dinnertime. My mom would cook from scratch every night, and then we would all sit around the dinner table and talk about our day." Jennie appreciated all the hard work and commitment it took from her parents to be able to maintain this special tradition for their family.

Her passion for nutrition and food didn't become clear until her late twenties when she was diagnosed with melanoma. "It was a very scary time in my life, but I knew that I could make better decisions for my overall health." She started learning about nutrition and holistic health, which led her to culinary school.

Jennie started her career in nutrition and food service after graduating from Johnson & Wales University in Charlotte, North Carolina. She spent over ten years working in the corporate food service management industry. She trained chefs across the country on how to write nutritious menus for clients of all ages from birth to retirement.

With a background in cheer and dance, Jennie has always enjoyed staying active. She continues to stay active now with E2M workouts and enjoys hiking with husband and twins. Jennie joined the E2M staff as one the chefs in November 2020 and has enjoyed teaching online cooking classes and being a part of every life that has been transformed by this program. "My heart's desire is to continue to educate others and share how to fuel your body, as well as to emphasize that healthy can be delicious!"

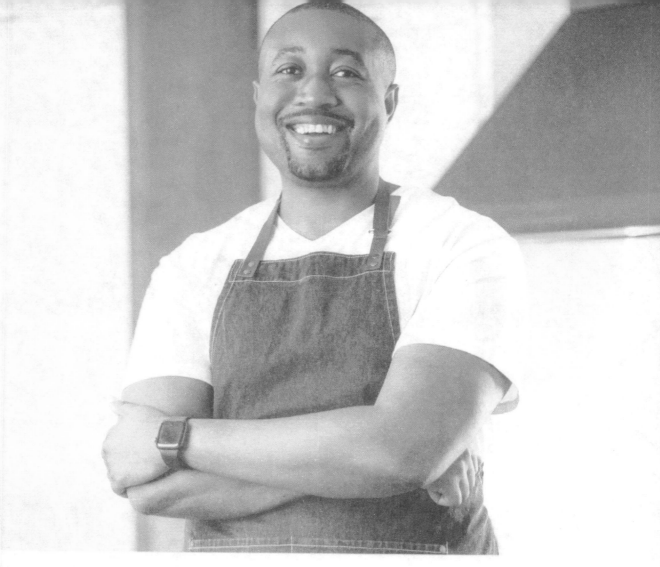

Andres Chaparro

Chef

Since he was young, Andres has always been involved with cooking. He started his career as an intern for a small bakery in his hometown. This gave him a little taste of the industry, which was all he needed to realize that he wanted to pursue a culinary career. After receiving formal training from Johnson & Wales University in Charlotte, North Carolina, he began working and gaining experience in kitchens from coast to coast. With over thirteen years of experience in the food service industry, he looks forward to bringing healthy cooking back to the main screen.

Andres first joined the E2M program in 2018 as a community member, which started his love of running. At the end of 2020, Andres transitioned to the E2M staff by providing weekly online cooking classes. Andres has enjoyed teaching countless E2M members how to make simple, healthy, and flavorful food.

e2mfitness.com

"Trust the Process™"

– JEFF WITHERSPOON

E2M™ Fitness
Success Stories

The jaw-dropping before and after photos of our clients are a direct result of following the E2M Fitness meal and exercise program.

The meal plan includes the recipes in all of our cookbooks written by the chefs of E2M Fitness.

Learning how to fuel your body with nutrient-dense proteins, vegetables, and healthy fats is the key to transitioning to a healthier lifestyle. With proper nutrition and exercise you can change your lifestyle! Healthy recipes and healthy habits lead to healthy living.

Success stories are shared throughout this cookbook. To learn more about the fitness program, please visit E2Mfitness.com

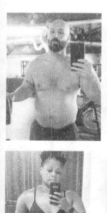
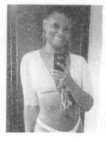
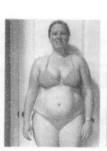
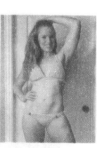
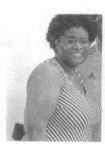
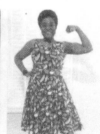
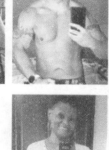
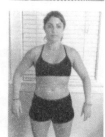
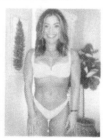
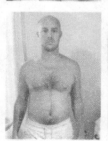
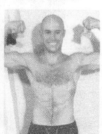
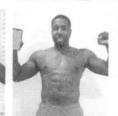
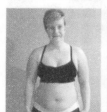
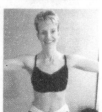
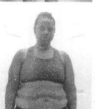

Meal Prep
Strategy

Why is meal prep so important?

Meal prep has become increasingly popular not only for those with busy schedules but also for those looking to eat healthier. Having healthy options readily available helps to manage cravings and to prevent you from making impulsive choices. Follow some of these time-saving strategies to help ditch the last-minute drive-thru and the extra expense of takeout.

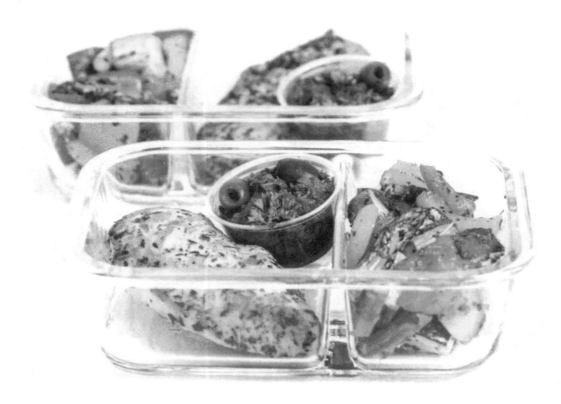

Meal Prep

Meal prep simply means preparing ingredients or whole meals in advance to save you time and set yourself up for success. It can be as simple as washing and chopping vegetables to be ready to cook on those busy weeknights. It can also be cooking and assembling entire meals that can be quickly heated and served for you or your whole family. Chopping vegetables or preparing meal components like your protein will save you time and energy, which we can all use more of during our busy seasons of life. Planned leftovers are another simple strategy to make sure you have healthy choices on hand. When you are preparing one recipe, simply make an extra serving to ensure you have another meal ready to take with you to work the next day. Spending a little extra time in the kitchen once or twice a week preparing your meal components is the key to a successful meal plan strategy.

Meal Prep Containers

Be sure to have plenty of storage containers with airtight lids to maintain quality and freshness. You can use glass or BPA-free plastic containers. For larger batch cooking and freezer meals, foil pans work great. Gallon-size ziplock bags and mason jars are ideal for storage. A vacuum sealer is a great option for preserving large amounts of prepared food, allowing food to remain safe for up to several months in the freezer.

Meal Prep Planning

Choose the recipes you would like to prepare for three to four days of meals. Try to select recipes that use similar ingredients to help reduce your grocery bill. Also check your local grocery store ads and farmers market to buy items that are on sale and seasonally available. You can use the **E2M Weekly Meal Planner** (see checklist pages) to track your recipes and make your grocery list based on your weekly meal plan. Then go to the store!

Grocery Shopping Tips:

1. Print and bring your weekly meal list.

2. Decide on which proteins you would like to prepare.

3. Choose two to three recipes you would like to make and select vegetables and fats to compliment the protein.

4. When shopping, stick to the perimeter of the store. Most of your fresh produce, proteins, and healthy fats are located on the outer perimeter of a grocery store. The inner aisles typically contain prepackaged foods that are not the most nutritious options available. Frozen and canned vegetables are also great options and another great way to meal prep.

5. Dry spices and herbs add loads of flavor to produce and proteins, so be sure to stock your spice cabinet with a variety of spices, including sea salt and black pepper!

6. Double-check food labels and ingredients to make sure there are no added sugars or ingredients that you cannot pronounce!

7. Only buy enough for three to four days so you do not waste food that may spoil quickly, such as fresh meats and produce.

Now you are ready to get in the kitchen and start cooking! Always be sure to read the entire recipe to ensure you are following the steps in order and you have all your ingredients. Enjoy prepping!

e2mfitness.com

Food
Safety

As you embark on your journey and getting back into the kitchen, it is important to know some basic food safety guidelines not only for yourself but also those you will be serving. Food safety plays a big part in your overall health journey. Germs can live in many conditions, so it is important to wash your produce, hands, utensils, and surfaces often while preparing food.

Wash Hands and Surfaces Often

- Never prep raw meat and vegetables on the same cutting board.
- Do not rinse or wash raw meat, seafood, or eggs.
- Did you know that the easiest way to prevent the spread of germs is to properly wash your hands? This is important and needs to be done any time that you are preparing different items in your kitchen. For example, you would need to wash your hands after you touch any uncooked proteins, ready-to-eat items, and vegetables.

- Properly washing your cutting boards with hot, soapy water after preparing each food item and before you go on to the next item is critical. This reduces the spread of germs and the risk of cross contamination.
- Chef Andres and Chef Jennie prefer to use separate cutting boards for proteins and vegetables. Plastic cutting boards are great for meat and wooden is best for vegetables and fruits. Wood boards are porous and can increase the likelihood of cross contamination.

Refrigerate and Store Properly

- As you start this journey into a healthier you, it may be tempting to overshop and pack your refrigerator with healthy items. It is important to not overstock your refrigerator. You need to allow adequate airflow to move throughout and keep the temperature around 40 degrees.
- Refrigerate perishable items like proteins within 2 hours of shopping.

- The freezer will be more efficient if kept full and if the top shelf is not crowded. Just like in the fridge, adequate airflow is critical.
- To prevent cross-contamination, do not store pre-cooked or plant-based "meat" next to raw meat. Wash and rinse all fresh produce before storing it in the fridge.
- Store raw meats and poultry at the bottom of the refrigerator to prevent cross-contamination with produce.

Temperature Control and Reheating

- Did you know there is a safe way to store your prepared meals and reheat them? The most important step of proper storage is not letting the meals stay out at room temperature for a long time before placing them in the refrigerator. When storing the meals in the refrigerator, place the food into smaller 1"-2" deep, airtight containers and ensure the lid is not tightly secured. This will allow steam from the food to

escape and adequately cool before placing the lid on and completing this process.
- When reheating your prepared meals, the Centers for Disease Control and Prevention recommends allowing food to reach to 165 degrees. When using a microwave, stir food halfway through cooking.
- By taking these steps, you are heading in the right direction regarding your food safety.

Cooking
Basics

Roasting and Baking
(325 to 450 degrees)

Roasting and baking are similar types of dry-heat cooking methods that use hot air to cook food. Roasting and baking at 325 to 450 degrees will brown the surface of the food, which will enhance the flavor. Roasting is a cooking method that can be done on sheet pans or roasting dishes. Chef Jennie prefers to roast on sheet pans covered with parchment paper to make for easy cleanup.

Roasting and baking are done in a standard oven. This technique cooks food evenly, at the same heat and at the same time. Roasting and baking require food be cooked uncovered to allow hot, dry air to circulate freely around the food. Proteins and vegetables can easily be cooked together with this technique. Be sure not to overcrowd your pan by putting food too close together. You want the air to circulate around the food to give it a nice crispy outside.

A meat thermometer is an extremely helpful tool to figure out the internal temperature of your protein and to know when it is a safe temperature for consuming. Cooking times can vary depending on equipment, so the use of a meat thermometer is the most exact way to find the internal temperature.

Cooking Tip: Prepare food for roasting and baking by cutting it into similar sizes so it cooks evenly.

Cooking Tip: Cover your sheet pan with parchment paper to clean up easily and to preserve the surface of the pans longer.

Broiling
(500 degrees)

Broiling is also a dry-heat cooking method that requires the food to be close to the heat source. This will cook the surface of the food quickly as well as brown the surface for more flavor. Chef Jennie and Chef Andres like to finish off dishes, especially chicken and fish, with two to three minutes under the broiler to enhance the flavors already used for the foods.

Cooking Tip: Stay close by when broiling; it only takes the broiler a few minutes before it can burn your food.

Grilling
(high heat)

Grilling simply means heating the food from below with high heat, whether using a gas, charcoal, or indoor grill. The food is typically only turned one time during the cooking process, giving the food the ever-so-desired grill marks. Grilling can also be achieved with a grill pan or grill grate that goes over a gas stove top. As with most cooking methods, it is important to heat the grill before adding the food and to make sure your grill grates are clean. Rather than oiling the pans or grates as you would with other cooking methods, oil your food directly when grilling.

Fish, chicken, vegetables, and fruit are better off being cooked at a lower temperature on the grill for a longer time.

Safety Tip: Always make sure the tools you use with a grill are specific for grilling and can stand up to high heat.

Sauté
(low to medium heat)

Sautéing is one of the most common ways to cook protein and vegetables at home. It is a quick cooking method that requires a little oil and a wide shallow pan. A helpful tip for sautéing food evenly is to not overcrowd your pan with too much food. Overcrowding can cause the heat to decrease and create steam that would end up steaming your food instead of sautéing it. To sauté food and make sure it cooks evenly, you can toss the food in the pan, then flip or move it around with a spatula. Think *Top Chef* or hibachi chef tricks!

It is important to allow your pan to heat up before adding a small amount of oil that has a high smoke point. Extra-virgin olive oil has a lower smoke point and will burn quickly. Allow the cooking oil to heat for a minute before adding the ingredients to the pan. Chef Jennie's and Chef Andres's recommended cooking oils are avocado oil and coconut oil spray.

Safety Tip: If using spray oils, please do not use over an open flame. Spray the pan prior to turning on a gas stove top.

Steaming and Boiling

Steaming and boiling are both low-fat cooking methods that do not require cooking oil. They do cook food at higher temperatures since the water needs to be boiling, but the indirect heat is what cooks the food during steaming. You will need a deep-sided pot and a steaming basket. Make sure to put enough water in the pot so that it doesn't evaporate out, but not too much to cause it to boil over. Most vegetables are excellent options for food for steaming and boiling.

Cast-Iron Skillet

Stove Top Cooking with Cast Iron: Cast iron's ability to absorb and distribute heat evenly makes it one of the best cooking vessels. Allow the cast-iron skillet to come to temperature by putting it over the heat for five to ten minutes to thoroughly heat. Once it reaches the desired temperature, it can consistently hold that temperature for an extended period of time, allowing you to cook your food evenly.

Chef Andres says, "When it comes to different cuts of meat, the best cooking process is a combination of both high- and low-temperature cooking methods." A cast-iron skillet is the perfect vessel for this method. Elevated temperatures sear and caramelize the outside, giving it the perfect outer crust to your protein. Chef Jennie loves to sear chicken and beef at a high heat to start and then finish off the cooking in the oven. Chef Jennie prefers to use her cast-iron skillet for most cooking methods!

Grilling with Cast Iron: Fish and vegetables can be challenging to grill since they are delicate. Using a cast-iron pan or griddle allows you to get that over-the-fire flavor without losing your food between the grates.

Safety and Care of Cast Iron: Cast-iron skillets require particular care but are worth it and will last for decades! Cleaning cast iron is easy. Avoid harsh detergents and soaps. If food is cooked onto the surface, add water and turn on the heat to bring it to a simmer. Use a wooden spoon to scrape the food from the pan and rinse. Once the skillet is clean and completely dry, rub it with a small amount of high-temperature oil—like avocado oil or coconut oil—to prevent rusting. This last step is the most important, according to Chef Jennie: don't forget to "season" your cast-iron skillet to prevent rust.

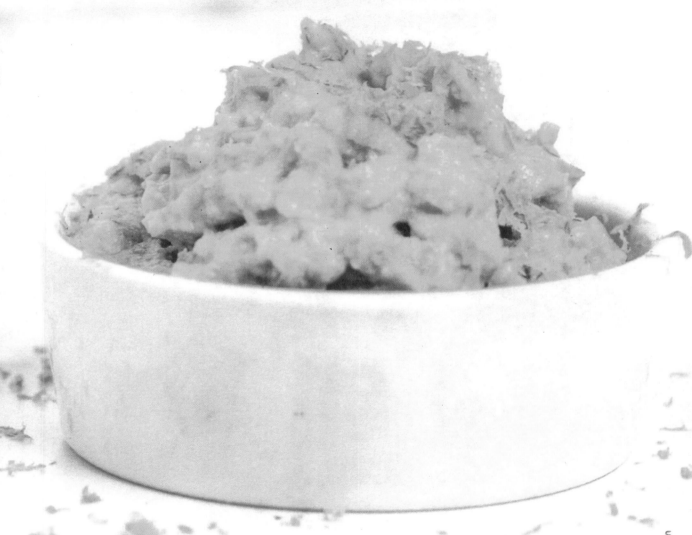

Meet the
Certified Trainers

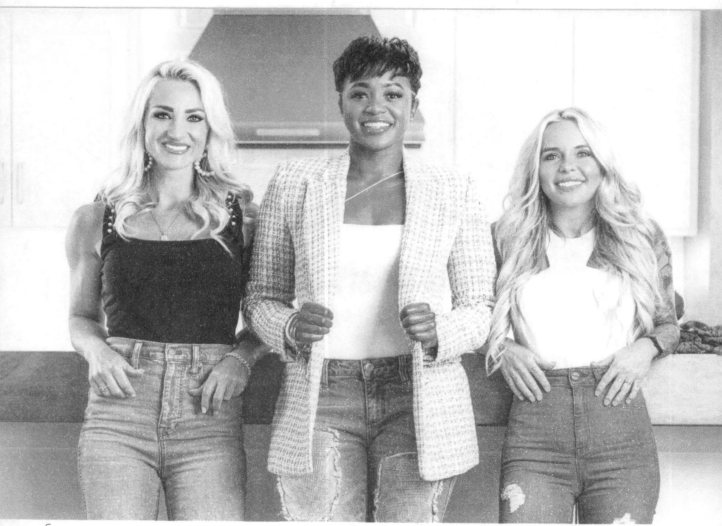

Mandy

"Fitness is
all-or-something,
not all-or-nothing"

Alicia

"Your GOAL is your destination!
Your ACTIONS are your vehicle!
CONSISTENCY and DISCIPLINE
are your fuel! Enjoy the journey
as much as the destination"

Whit

"The body
achieves what
the mind believes"

Suggested
Kitchen Tools

Measuring Tools

Digital scale

Measuring cups

Measuring spoons

Meat thermometer

Utensils

Tongs

Rubber and metal spatulas

Wooden spoon

Zester/Microplane

Sharp knife

Vegetable peeler

Can opener

Citrus juicer

Plastic cutting board
(best for proteins)

Wood cutting board
(best for fruits and vegetables)

Cooking Vessels

Cast-iron skillet

Sauté pan

Sheet pans

Roasting pans

Grill (gas or charcoal)

Grill pan for indoor grilling

Air fryer

Steaming basket

Other
Suggested Items

Heat-resistant gloves or towels

Oven mitts

Salad spinner

Colander

E2M apron

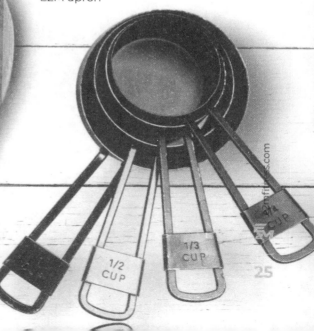

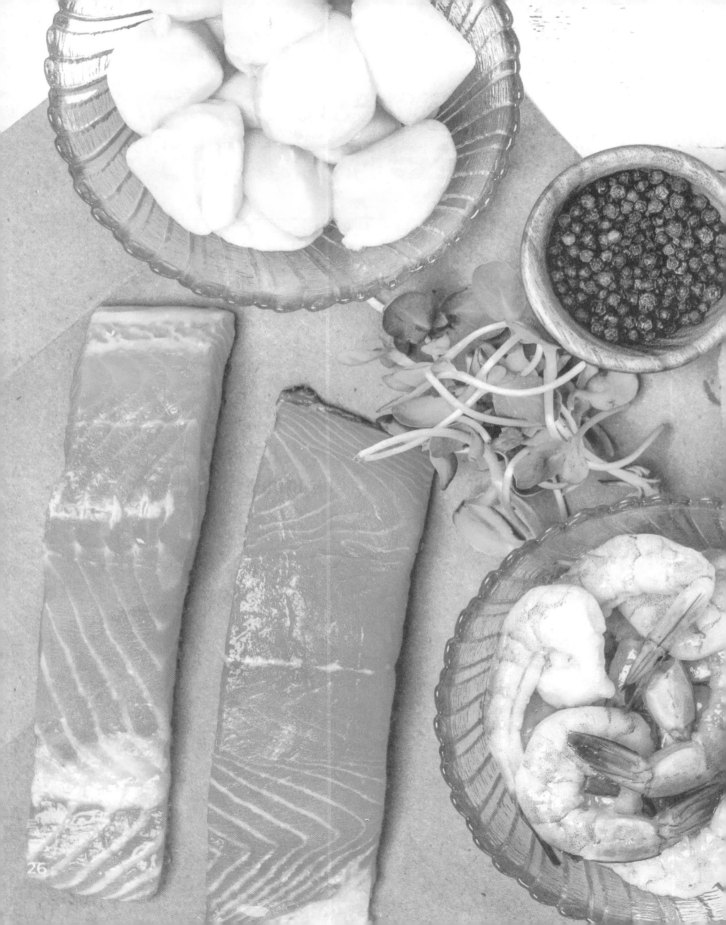

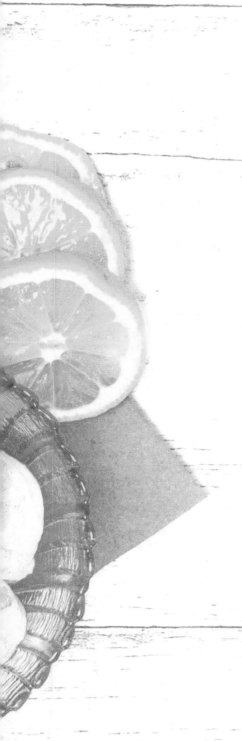

Seafood

⧗ Success Stories

Titus I., Charlotte, NC

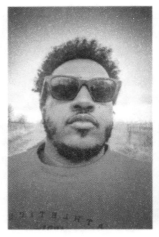 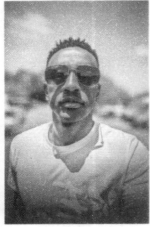

Rounds	Age	Weight Loss
5	39	101

I wanted to become the very best version of myself for my family. I have a four-year-old son that I want to have the energy to keep up with now and as he gets older.

What were you hoping to gain from your E2M experience?
I have already gained so much from my E2M experience, so I just hope that I can continue to meet wonderful people in the E2M community, continue to inspire others, and continue being inspired by others.

Non-Scale Victory (NSV)!
I beat hypertension and obesity!

Samantha M., Gloucester Township, NJ

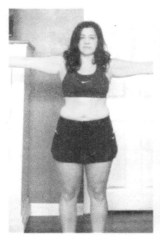 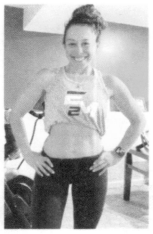

Rounds	Age	Weight Loss
4	49	17

I'm a single mom with two kids and three jobs, along with a house to care for. My health was my last priority and E2M fitness has changed that. It's made me a better mom, employee, and overall happier person. The E2M program also introduced me to the best friends I've ever had.

What does the E2M community mean to you?
It means amazing trainers, support I've never seen in any program before, and structure that I needed.

Non-Scale Victory (NSV)!
No more antidepressants. I have so much more energy. I'm happier, stronger, and more organized.

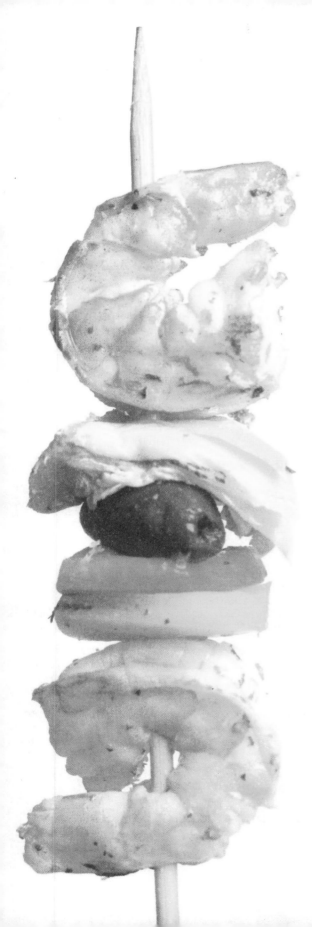

Shrimp

Southern Shrimp
and Creamy Cauliflower

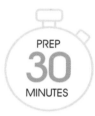

PREP
30
MINUTES

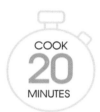

COOK
20
MINUTES

SERVES
4

Ingredients

Shrimp:
- 2 pounds (31/35) shrimp, fresh or frozen, peeled and deveined
- 1 tablespoon minced garlic
- 1 lemon, zested and juiced
- 2 tablespoons Seafood Spice Blend (see page 127)
- Cooking spray
- 1 tablespoon rice vinegar
- 1 red bell pepper, seeded and sliced
- 1 green bell pepper, seeded and sliced
- Fresh chopped parsley (for garnish)

Cauliflower:
- 2 cauliflower heads, cut into florets
- ¼ teaspoon sea salt
- ⅛ teaspoon black pepper

Prep

1. If using frozen shrimp, thaw in a colander under running water.

2. Prepare the shrimp in a large bowl by first combining the minced garlic, lemon zest (reserving some lemon zest for garnish), and 2 tablespoons Seafood Spice Blend; mix thoroughly. Add the shrimp to the bowl; toss to coat evenly. Refrigerate for 30 minutes.

Cook

3. In a large pot, bring water to a boil; add the cauliflower pieces and boil on high until tender, about 20 minutes. Drain and let cool. Puree with a food processor or immersion blender until smooth. Season with salt and pepper.

4. To cook the shrimp, spray a pan with cooking spray. Sauté the shrimp in batches over medium heat until the shrimp turn pink, 2 to 3 minutes on each side. The shrimp will look like the letter C when raw and the letter G when fully cooked. Note that it is best to cook the shrimp in batches.

5. After the last batch of shrimp is cooked and set aside, pour the vinegar into the pan over medium heat to release any cooked-on seasonings; scrape with a wooden spoon. Add the sliced peppers to the pan; sauté for 5 to 8 minutes, or until tender.

Serve

6. Spoon the pureed cauliflower into a bowl, top with sautéed peppers and shrimp. Garnish with chopped parsley, lemon juice, and the remaining lemon zest.

Notes:
If you like spicy, include a dash of your favorite hot sauce or crushed red pepper to add some extra spice to the dish.

e2mfitness.com

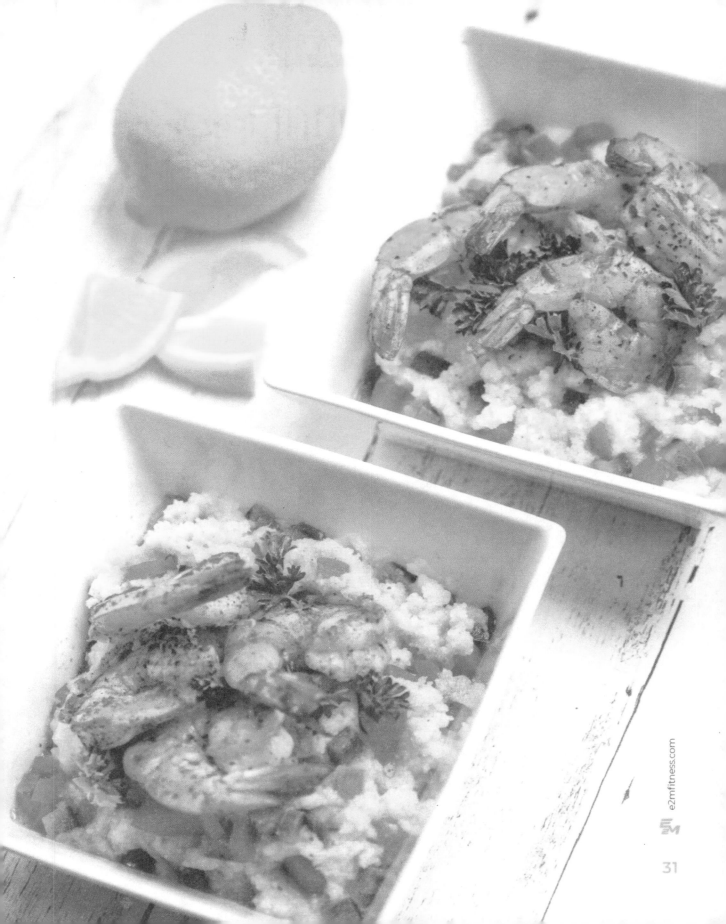

BBQ Shrimp
with Zucchini and Peppers

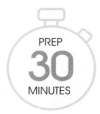

PREP
30
MINUTES

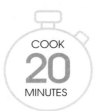

COOK
20
MINUTES

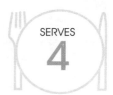

SERVES
4

Ingredients

Shrimp and Vegetables:
- 2 pounds (31/35) shrimp, fresh or frozen, peeled and deveined
- Cooking spray
- 1 tablespoon rice vinegar
- 3 zucchini, sliced (peeled if preferred)

- 2 red bell peppers, seeded and sliced
- 2 avocados, peeled and diced
- 1½ teaspoons chopped fresh parsley (for garnish)
- Spice blend (see below for recipe)

Spice Blend:
- ½ teaspoon chili powder
- ½ teaspoon ground garlic
- ½ teaspoon dried smoked paprika
- ½ teaspoon ground cumin
- ¼ teaspoon sea salt
- ⅛ teaspoon black pepper

- ¼ teaspoon chipotle seasoning (or more, depending on desired spice level)
- 1 tablespoon ground mustard or Dijon mustard
- 1 tablespoon water

Prep

1. If using frozen shrimp, thaw in a colander under running water.
2. Prepare the spice blend in a large bowl by combining the chili powder, garlic, smoked paprika, cumin, chipotle seasoning, sea salt, black pepper, mustard, and water; mix thoroughly. Add the shrimp to the bowl; toss to coat evenly. Refrigerate for 30 minutes.

Cook

3. Heat the cooking oil in a skillet or large pan over medium heat. Add the seasoned shrimp; sauté the shrimp in batches until the shrimp turn pink. Cook for 2 to 3 minutes on each side. The shrimp will look like the letter C when raw and the letter G when fully cooked. Note that it is best to cook the shrimp in batches.
   Air fryer option: Cook the shrimp for 5 minutes at 300 degrees.
4. After the last batch of shrimp is cooked and set aside, pour the rice vinegar into the pan over medium heat to release any cooked-on seasonings; sc with a wooden spoon. Add the sliced zucchini and sliced red bell pepper. sauté for 5 to 8 minutes, or until tender.

Serve

5. Plate the zucchini and red bell peppers; top with shrimp and diced avocado. Garnish with fresh parsley.

Pineapple Shrimp
Stir-Fry

Ingredients

Shrimp:
- 2 pounds (31/35) shrimp, fresh or frozen, peeled and deveined
- Cooking spray
- 1 tablespoon vinegar
- 1 cup shredded carrots
- 1 cup diced red bell peppers
- 1 cup diced mushrooms (cremini or baby bella)

- 2 cups shredded cabbage or coleslaw
- 1 cup diced pineapple
- ½ cup chopped peanuts
- 1 lime, zested and juiced
- 2 tablespoons chopped cilantro (for garnish)
- Stir-fry marinade

Stir-Fry Marinade:
- 1 tablespoon olive oil
- 1 tablespoon rice vinegar
- 1 tablespoon dried basil
- 1 tablespoon ground garlic

- 1½ teaspoons ground ginger
- 1 lime, zested and juiced
- ¼ teaspoon sea salt
- ⅛ teaspoon black pepper

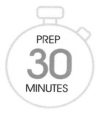

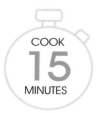

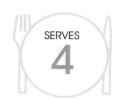

Prep

1. If using frozen shrimp, thaw in a colander under running water.

2. Prepare the stir-fry marinade in a large bowl by combining the olive oil, rice vinegar, basil, garlic, ginger, lime zest, lime juice, sea salt, and black pepper; mix thoroughly. Add the shrimp to the bowl; toss to coat evenly. Refrigerate for 30 minutes.

Cook

3. Spray a pan with cooking spray. Sauté the shrimp in batches over medium heat until the shrimp turn pink, 2 to 3 minutes on each side. The shrimp will look like the letter C when raw and the letter G when fully cooked. Note that it is best to cook the shrimp in batches.
   Air fryer option: Cook the shrimp for 5 minutes at 300 degrees.

4. After the last batch of shrimp is cooked and set aside, pour the vinegar into the pan over medium heat to release any cooked-on seasonings; scrape with a wooden spoon. Add the carrots, diced red bell peppers, mushrooms, and shredded cabbage to the pan; sauté for 5 to 8 minutes, or until tender.

Serve

5. Divide the vegetables between the plates; top with shrimp, pineapple, and chopped peanuts. Garnish with fresh cilantro and lime zest.

e2mfitness.com

Oven-Roasted
Greek Shrimp Skewers

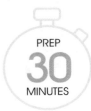

PREP
30
MINUTES

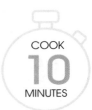

COOK
10
MINUTES

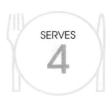

SERVES
4

Ingredients

Shrimp:

- 10 wooden or reusable metal skewers
- 2 pounds (31/35) shrimp, fresh or frozen, peeled and deveined
- 1 large red bell pepper, seeded and large dice
- 1 large green bell pepper, seeded and large dice
- 4 handfuls of spring mix
- 1 can (14 ounces) artichoke hearts, drained, quartered
- 1 can (6 ounces) whole black olives, drained
- 1 lemon, zest and juice
- Fresh parsley (for garnish)
- Cooking spray
- Herb blend (see below for recipe)

Herb Blend:

- 1½ teaspoons dried oregano
- 1½ teaspoons dried basil
- 1 teaspoon ground garlic
- 1 lemon, zested and juiced
- ¼ teaspoon sea salt
- ⅛ teaspoon black pepper
- 2 tablespoons fresh chopped parsley
- 1 tablespoon olive oil

Prep

1. Soak the wooden skewers in water for 30 minutes prior to using, in order to prevent splintering and burning. If the shrimp is frozen, thaw in a colander under running water.

2. Prepare the herb blend in a large bowl by combining the oregano, basil, garlic, lemon zest, lemon juice, sea salt, black pepper, parsley, and olive oil; mix thoroughly. Add the shrimp, diced red bell peppers, diced green bell peppers, diced artichoke hearts, and olives; toss to coat evenly. Refrigerate for 30 minutes.

3. Preheat the oven to 400 degrees. Line a sheet pan with parchment paper or spray with cooking spray. Assemble the skewers by alternating vegetables and shrimp until each skewer is full.

Cook

4. Put the skewers on the pan. Bake for 7 to 8 minutes, or until the shrimp turn pink. The shrimp will look like the letter C when raw and the letter G when fully cooked. Note that it is best to cook the shrimp in batches. Squeeze fresh lemon juice over warm shrimp.

Serve

5. Arrange the skewers on plates over spring mix and garnish with fresh parsley. This is a great dish that's easy to serve and for entertaining a large crowd.

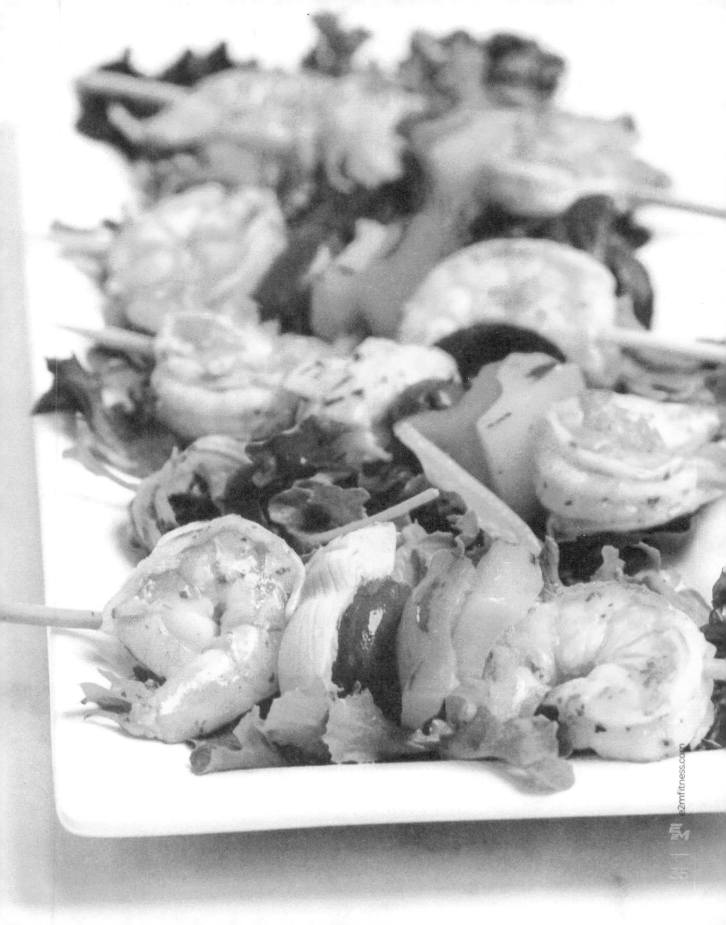

E2M Success Stories

Jon R., KENTWOOD, MI

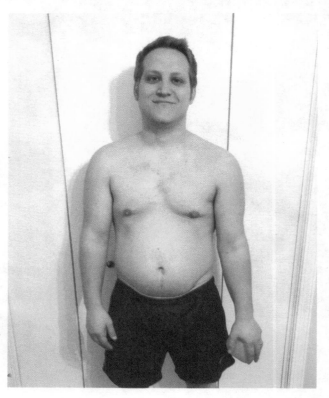 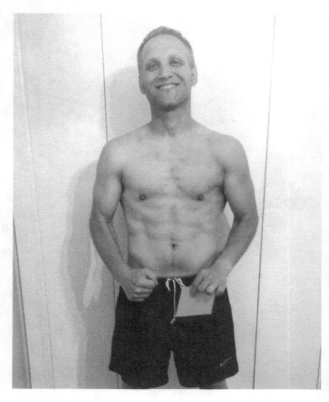

Rounds	Age	Weight Loss
1	36	40

As a father of five, I got into a routine of convenience, and my personal health was not important to me. The E2M program fits around my kids' schedules. The flexibility allowed me to regain my health, work out with my wife, and still be 100 percent involved with my kids' activities.

What did you want to change about your lifestyle?
The unhealthy eating and drinking habits were the biggest changes I wanted to make. Every day I was drinking over eighty ounces of energy drinks or soda, eating five to ten bite-size candy bars, and regularly eating fast food for convenience.

What is your favorite type of workout?
The circuits are my favorite workouts. They're incredibly challenging, offer a wide variety of exercises, and allow you to get to know the coaches' personalities.

Chili-Lime Shrimp
and Vegetables

Ingredients

- 2 pounds (31/35) shrimp, fresh or frozen, peeled and deveined
- 2½ tablespoons Chili-Lime Seasoning (see page 120)
- Cooking spray
- 6 cups chopped spinach

- 2 red bell peppers, seeded and thinly sliced
- 2 green bell peppers, seeded and thinly sliced
- 2 avocado, peeled and diced
- 1 lime, zest and juice
- Hot sauce - to taste

Prep

1. For the Chili-Lime Seasoning, combine all the ingredients and mix well; store in an airtight container.

2. If the shrimp is frozen, thaw in a colander under running water. Toss the shrimp in 2 tablespoons of the Chili-Lime Seasoning.

Cook

3. Heat a pan over medium heat; spray the pan with cooking spray. Sauté the shrimp in batches over medium heat until the shrimp turn pink, 2 to 3 minutes on each side. The shrimp will look like the letter C when raw and the letter G when fully cooked. Note that it is best to cook the shrimp in batches. Remove the shrimp from the pan. Squeeze juice of one lime into pan and use a wooden spoon to scrape the bottom. Add the red peppers, green peppers, and sauté for 3 to 5 minutes, or until tender. Remove and add the spinach in batches until it wilts down.

4. In a small bowl, toss the diced avocado with ½ teaspoon of the Chili-Lime Seasoning.

Serve

5. Plate the vegetables and top with diced avocado and sautéed shrimp.

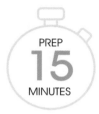

PREP
15
MINUTES

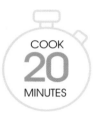

COOK
20
MINUTES

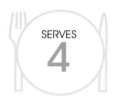

SERVES
4

Meal prep idea:
Store the shrimp and cooked vegetables together in an airtight container; refrigerate for up to three days. Assemble the spinach and avocado when ready to eat.

e2mfitness.com

Buffalo Shrimp
with Sautéed Kale

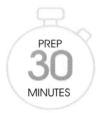

PREP
30
MINUTES

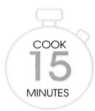

COOK
15
MINUTES

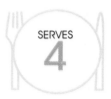

SERVES
4

Ingredients

Shrimp and Kale:
- 2 pounds (31/35) shrimp, fresh or frozen, peeled and deveined
- 1½ teaspoons ground garlic
- 2 teaspoons dried smoked paprika
- 2 teaspoons chili powder
- Cooking spray
- 1 tablespoon apple cider vinegar
- 2 pounds chopped kale
- 2 avocados, peeled and diced

Shrimp Hot Sauce:
- 3 tablespoons hot sauce
- 1 tablespoon apple cider vinegar
- ½ tablespoon olive oil

Prep

1. If using frozen shrimp, thaw in a colander under running water.
2. In a large bowl, combine the garlic, paprika, and chili powder; mix thoroughly. Add the shrimp to the bowl; toss to coat evenly. Refrigerate for 30 minutes.

Cook

3. Heat the skillet or large pan over medium heat. Spray pan with cooking oil. Add the seasoned shrimp; sauté the shrimp in batches until the shrimp turn pink. Cook for 2 to 3 minutes on each side. The shrimp will look like the letter C when raw and the letter G when fully cooked. Note that it is best to cook the shrimp in batches.
4. Combine the hot sauce, apple cider vinegar, and olive oil in a large bowl; add the cooked shrimp and toss to coat evenly.
5. Pour 1 tablespoon apple cider vinegar into the pan over medium heat to release any cooked-on seasonings; scrape with a wooden spoon. Add the kale and sauté for 5 to 8 minutes, or until the leaves are tender and slightly wilted.

Serve

6. Plate the sautéed kale; top each portion with shrimp and diced avocado

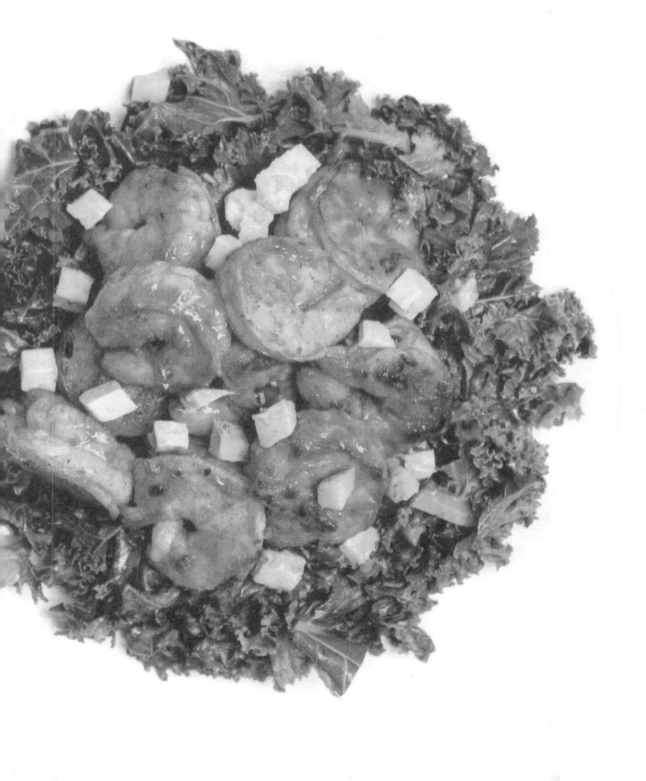

Peri Peri Shrimp
with Green Beans

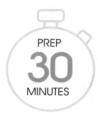

PREP
30
MINUTES

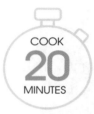

COOK
20
MINUTES

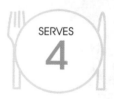

SERVES
4

Ingredients

- 2 pounds (31/35) shrimp, fresh or frozen, peeled and deveined
- 2 tablespoons Peri Peri Spice Blend (see page 121)
- 1 lime, zested and juiced
- Cooking spray

- 1 cup sliced bella mushrooms
- 2 bags (12 ounces each) frozen green beans
- 1 teaspoon Peri Peri Spice Blend (more as desired)

Prep

1. For the Peri Peri Spice Blend, whisk together all the ingredients in a small bowl. Transfer to an airtight container or jar.

2. If the shrimp is frozen, thaw in a colander under running water.

3. In a large bowl, combine the 2 tablespoons Peri Peri Spice Blend, lime zest, and lime juice. Add the shrimp to the bowl; toss to coat evenly. Refrigerate for 30 minutes or until ready to cook.

Cook

4. Heat a large skillet over medium heat and spray with cooking spray. Add the seasoned shrimp; sauté the shrimp in batches until the shrimp turn pink. Cook for 2 to 3 minutes on each side. The shrimp will look like the letter C when raw and the letter G when fully cooked. Note that it is best to cook the shrimp in batches. Remove shrimp from pan.

5. Spray more cooking oil if needed; add the sliced mushrooms to the pan. Stirring frequently, cook until the mushrooms are soft, about 3 minutes. Add the frozen green beans and toss to coat them in the oil and spices; cook for another 2 to 3 minutes. Add the 1 teaspoon Peri Peri Spice Blend, or more if desired; stir to combine and let everything cook for about 3 minutes.

Serve

6. Plate the mushrooms and greens beans; top with shrimp.

Sheet-Pan
Mediterranean Shrimp

Ingredients

- 2 pounds (31/35) shrimp, fresh or frozen, peeled and deveined
- 2 teaspoons olive oil, divided
- 2½ tablespoons Mediterranean Spice Blend, divided (see page 120)
- 2 bunches fresh asparagus, chopped
- 2 cups sliced mushrooms
- 2 red bell peppers, seeded and sliced
- 1 can (14 ounces) artichoke hearts, drained, cut into quarters
- 1 cup Kalamata olives, drained
- 1 lemon, zest and juice
- 2 tablespoons chopped fresh basil

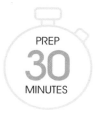

PREP
30
MINUTES

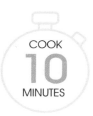

COOK
10
MINUTES

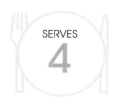

SERVES
4

Prep

1. For the Mediterranean Spice Blend, combine all the ingredients and mix well; store in an airtight container.

2. If using frozen shrimp, thaw in a colander under running water.

3. Preheat the oven to 400 degrees. Line a sheet pan with parchment paper or spray with cooking spray.

4. In a large bowl, combine the shrimp, 1 teaspoon of the olive oil, and 1 tablespoon of the Mediterranean Spice Blend.

5. In a separate bowl, mix 1 teaspoon of the olive oil in a large bowl with 1½ tablespoons of the Mediterranean Spice Blend. Add the chopped asparagus, sliced red bell peppers, sliced mushrooms, quartered artichoke hearts, and olives. Toss to combine and spread over the parchment-lined sheet pan. Arrange the shrimp on top of the mixed vegetables. Zest the lemon over the whole sheet pan; thinly slice the lemon into rounds, layering them over the shrimp and vegetables.

Cook

6. Bake at 400 degrees for 10 minutes, or until the shrimp turn pink and look like the letter G.

Serve

7. Plate the vegetables and top with shrimp. Sprinkle with chopped fresh basil and lemon juice.

Chimichurri Shrimp
Lettuce Tacos

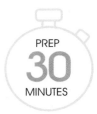

PREP
30
MINUTES

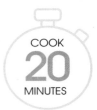

COOK
20
MINUTES

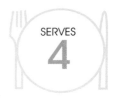

SERVES
4

Ingredients

Shrimp and Vegetables:
- 2 pounds (31/35) shrimp, fresh or frozen, peeled and deveined
- Lettuce leaves (bibb lettuce or romaine work best)
- 2 red or green bell peppers, seeded and thinly sliced
- ½ red onion, thinly sliced
- 2 avocados, peeled and diced
- Chimichurri sauce (recipe below)
- Cooking spray

Chimichurri Sauce:
- ½ cup chopped fresh parsley leaves
- ½ cup chopped fresh cilantro leaves
- ½ cup extra-virgin olive oil
- ¼ cup red wine vinegar
- 1½ teaspoons ground garlic
- ½ teaspoon dried oregano
- ⅛ teaspoon crushed red pepp‹

Prep

1. If using frozen shrimp, thaw in a colander under running water.

2. For the chimichurri sauce, combine the ingredients in a food processor; blend until smooth. Reserve 3 tablespoons of sauce. Transfer the remaining chimichurri sauce to a large bowl, add the shrimp, and toss to coat evenly. Marinate in the refrigerator for at least 30 minutes.

Cook

3. Heat a pan over medium heat; spray the pan with cooking spray. Sauté the shrimp in batches over medium heat until the shrimp turn pink, 2 to 3 minutes on each side. The shrimp will look like the letter C when raw and the letter G when fully cooked. Note that it is best to cook the shrimp in batches. Remove the shrimp from the pan. Add peppers and onions to the pan and sauté for 3 to 5 minutes, or until tender.

Serve

4. Place a large lettuce leaf on each plate; put the shrimp and sautéed onions and red bell peppers on the lettuce; top with diced avocado and the remaining chimichurri sauce.

Meal prep idea:
Store the shrimp and vegetables together in an airtight container; put the lettuce leaves in a ziplock bag with a paper towel. Refrigerate for up to three days. Assemble when ready to eat.

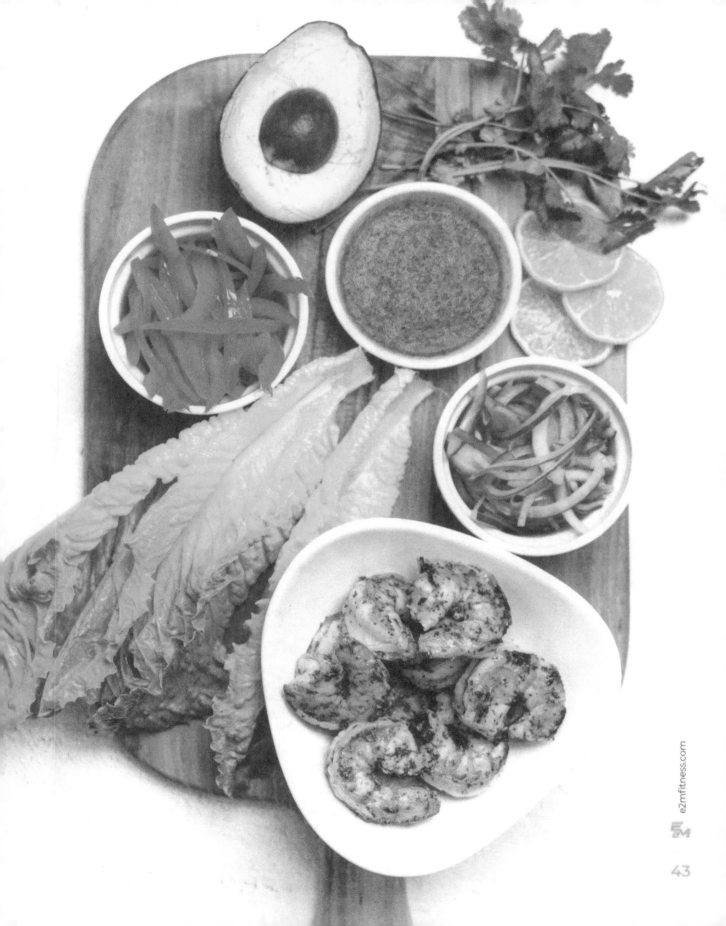

⧖ Success Stories

Krista T., Mattoon, IL

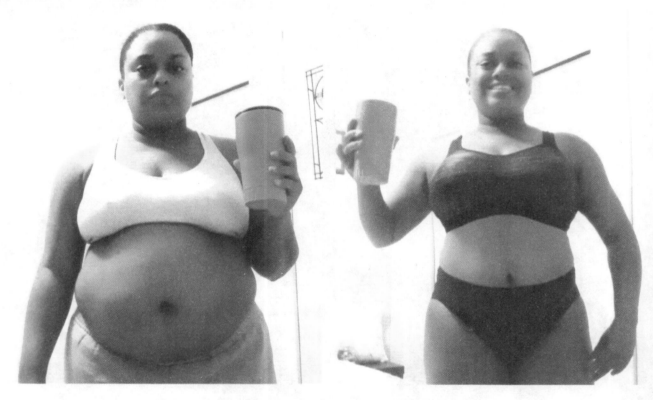

Rounds	Age	Weight Loss
1	**42**	**16**

I joined the E2M program because I wanted to improve my overall health since I suffer from polycystic ovary syndrome, depression and anxiety, and I'm prediabetic. I've since been able to scale back on medications and my lab work has shown significant improvement by lowering my A1C!

How has E2M fitness changed your life?
The E2M program has ABSOLUTELY changed my life! I feel purposeful and life is worth living even more!

What is your favorite type of workout?
I am a huge fan of the Pilates and yoga workouts.

Thai Shrimp
with Sautéed Vegetables

Ingredients

Shrimp:

- 2 pounds (31/35) shrimp, fresh or frozen, peeled and deveined
- Cooking spray

- 2 tablespoons Thai Spice Blend (see page 127)
- 2 limes, zested and juiced

Sautéed vegetables:

- 2 red bell peppers, seeded and diced
- 2 (8-ounce) packages of shredded cabbage mix
- 1 lime, juiced
- 1 tablespoon Thai Spice Blend

- ¼ teaspoon crushed red pepper (optional)
- Handful of fresh cilantro, chopped, divided
- ¼ cup cashews, chopped

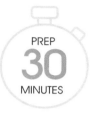

PREP
30
MINUTES

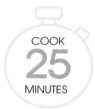

COOK
25
MINUTES

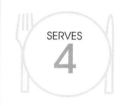

SERVES
4

Prep

1. For the Thai Spice Blend, combine all the ingredients and mix well; store in an airtight container.

2. If using frozen shrimp, thaw in a colander under running water.

3. In a large bowl, combine 1 tablespoon of the Thai Spice Blend, the lime zest, and lime juice; mix thoroughly. Add the shrimp to the bowl; toss to coat evenly. Refrigerate for at least 30 minutes or until ready to cook.

Cook

4. Heat a large skillet over medium heat and spray with cooking spray. Cook the shrimp in batches over medium heat until the shrimp turn pink, 2 to 3 minutes on each side. The shrimp will look like the letter C when raw and the letter G when fully cooked. Note that it is best to cook the shrimp in batches.

5. Return the skillet to medium heat. Squeeze the juice of 1 lime into pan and use a wooden spoon to scrape the bottom of the pan. Spray more cooking oil if needed; add the diced red bell peppers to the pan. Stirring frequently, cook until the peppers are soft, about 3 minutes. Add the shredded cabbage, 1 tablespoon of Thai Spice blend, and optional red pepper for heat. and toss to coat in oil and spices; cook for another 2 to 3 minutes.

6. Stir to combine and let everything cook for about 3 to 5 minutes. Add half of the chopped cilantro and remove from the heat.

Serve

7. Plate the sautéed vegetables; top with the shrimp and garnish with the remaining cilantro and the cashews.

Chili-Lime Shrimp
with Cilantro Cauliflower Rice

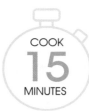

PREP
30
MINUTES

COOK
15
MINUTES

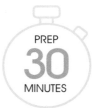

SERVES
4

Ingredients

Shrimp:

- 2 pounds (31/35) shrimp, fresh or frozen, peeled and deveined
- 2 teaspoons dried smoked paprika
- 1 teaspoon ground garlic
- 1 teaspoon black pepper
- 1 teaspoon dried oregano
- ½ teaspoon ground cayenne pepper
- 2 teaspoons sea salt
- 2 teaspoons chili powder
- 2 teaspoons olive oil
- 1 lime, zested
- Cooking spray

Cilantro Cauliflower Rice:

- ½ cup chopped mushrooms
- 1 bell pepper, diced
- 1 teaspoon ground garlic
- 1 teaspoon ground chili powder
- 1 green jalapeño, seeded and sliced (optional)
- 8 cups riced cauliflower (frozen or shelf stable)
- 4 tablespoons water
- 1 teaspoon sea salt (more as needed)
- 1 lime, zest and juice
- ½ cup chopped fresh cilantro, divided

Prep

1. If using frozen shrimp, thaw in a colander under running water.

2. In a large bowl, prepare a marinade for the shrimp by combining the smoked paprika, garlic, black pepper, oregano, cayenne pepper, sea salt, chili powder, olive oil, and the zest from one lime; mix thoroughly. Add the shrimp to the bowl; toss to coat evenly. Marinate for 30 minutes or until ready to cook.

Cook

3. To cook the shrimp, spray a pan with cooking oil. Sauté the shrimp in batches over medium heat until the shrimp turn pink, 2 to 3 minutes on each side. The shrimp will look like the letter C when raw and the letter G when fully cooked. Note that it is best to cook the shrimp in batches.

4. In the same pan, add more cooking spray, add the chopped mushrooms and diced bell pepper; sauté over medium heat until they become soft and translucent, 4 to 5 minutes. Add the garlic, chili powder, and optional jalapeño; cook for another minute, stirring the whole time.

5. Add the cauliflower to the skillet; stir well to mix everything together. Stir in the salt, lime zest, and half the cilantro. Turn the heat up to high and cook for another minute. The high heat will draw out excess moisture in the cauliflower, so it will not get mushy. Remove from heat and stir in the remaining cilantro.

Serve

6. Plate the cilantro cauliflower rice and top with the seasoned shrimp. Garnish with fresh lime zest and juice.

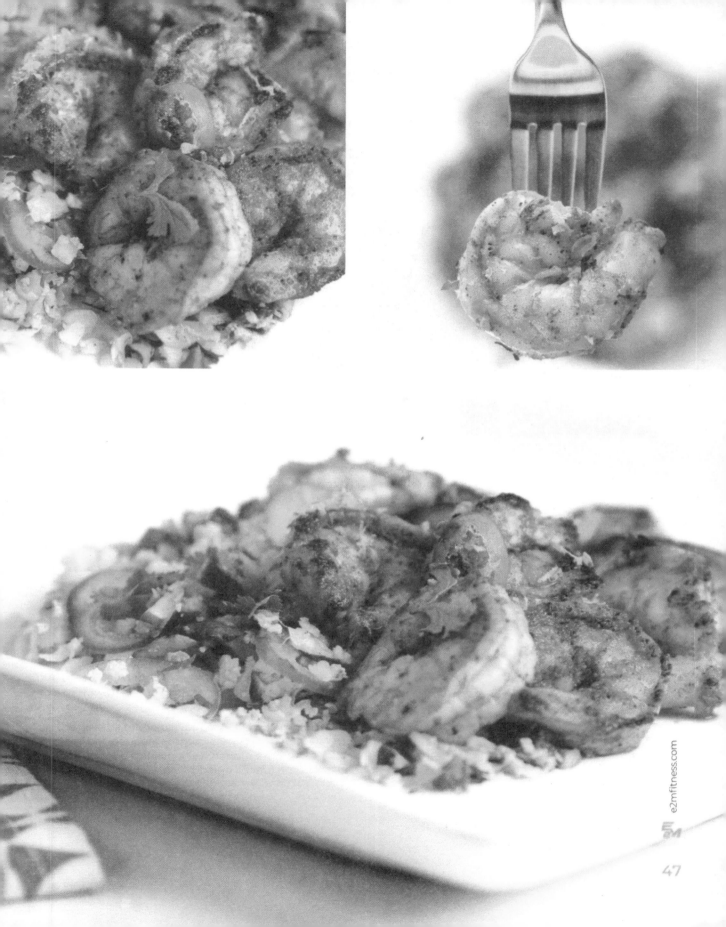

≡M Success Stories

Alexander M., Goose Creek, SC

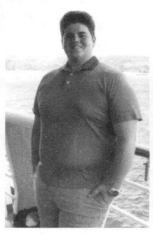 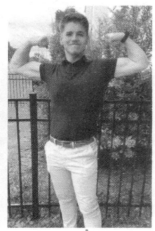

Rounds	Age	Weight Loss
6	22	120

I've been obese for as long as I can remember. I've had many health problems associated with the weight and I was constantly worried about the longevity of my life. Now I have the skills to maintain a healthy lifestyle forever. The confidence I've gained from achieving what seemed impossible has seeped into other aspects of my life and has made me a better person. My next step is working on getting more toned.

What were you hoping to gain from your E2M experience?
The skills to get the weight off and KEEP the weight off.

Allison J., MD St. Louis, MO

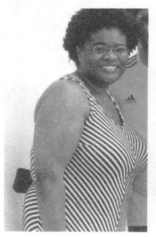 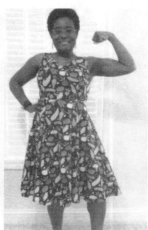

Rounds	Age	Weight Loss
8	41	75

The E2M fitness program has completely changed my relationship with food. I now see food as fuel and have developed the discipline to enjoy treats in moderation. It has also helped me recover from cancer treatment. Thanks to the program, I am stronger mentally and physically, more confident, and my goals and values for health and wellness are in alignment with my actions.

Non-Scale Victory (NSV)!
My chemotherapy-induced cardiomyopathy has improved from 45 percent to 56 percent.

What is your favorite type of workout?
Zumba (aka Church of Zumba).

e2mfitness.com

≡M

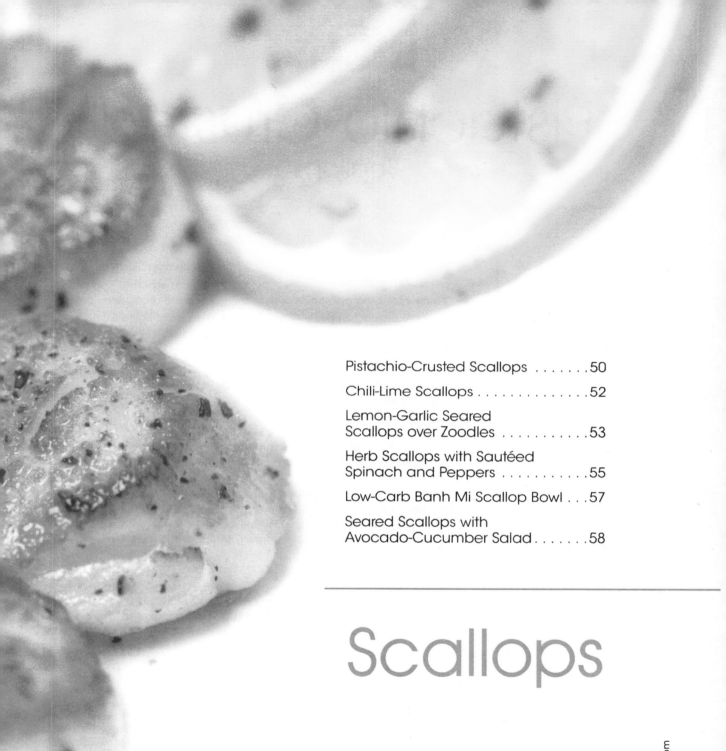

Scallops

Pistachio-Crusted
Scallops

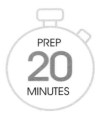

PREP
20
MINUTES

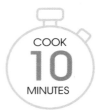

COOK
10
MINUTES

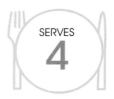

SERVES
4

Ingredients

- *2 pounds sea scallops (20 to 30 per pound)
- 2 ounces shelled pistachios
- 1 lemon, zested
- ½ teaspoon black pepper
- 1 teaspoon chives
- Cooking spray
- ½ teaspoon fresh thyme, finely chopped
- 1 tablespoon extra-virgin olive oil
- 1 bunch asparagus spears, chopped on a bias
- 6 handfuls spinach
- ½ teaspoon sea salt
- ⅛ teaspoon black pepper

Prep

1. *If using frozen scallops, allow them to thaw overnight in the refrigerator; do not thaw at room temperature. Use paper towels to pat dry the thawed or fresh scallops.

2. Put the pistachios in a small food processor; pulse until they resemble crumbs. Transfer the pistachio crumbs to a shallow dish, and stir in the lemon zest. Set aside. Season the scallops on all sides with the remaining ½ teaspoon of coarse salt, black pepper, chives, and chopped thyme.

Cook

3. Heat a large pan to medium-high heat. When the pan begins to smoke, spray the pan with cooking oil; put the seasoned scallops in the pan. Do not overcrowd the pan, which will cause the scallops to steam; it's best to allow space between and cook in batches. Sauté the scallops until browned, 2 to 3 minutes; flip and cook on the other side until the scallops are slightly firm, 1 to 2 minutes.

4. Use tongs to transfer the scallops to the dish with the pistachio crumbs; turn and toss the scallops until they are coated on all sides.

5. Heat the olive oil in the skillet over medium-high heat. Add the chopped asparagus and cook for 1 to 2 minutes. Remove the pan from the heat, add the spinach, and mix. Remove the spinach when it begins to wilt but be careful not to over cook it. Season with salt and pepper to taste.

Serve

6. Plate the sautéed asparagus and spinach on the plates, and top with the pistachio-crusted scallops.

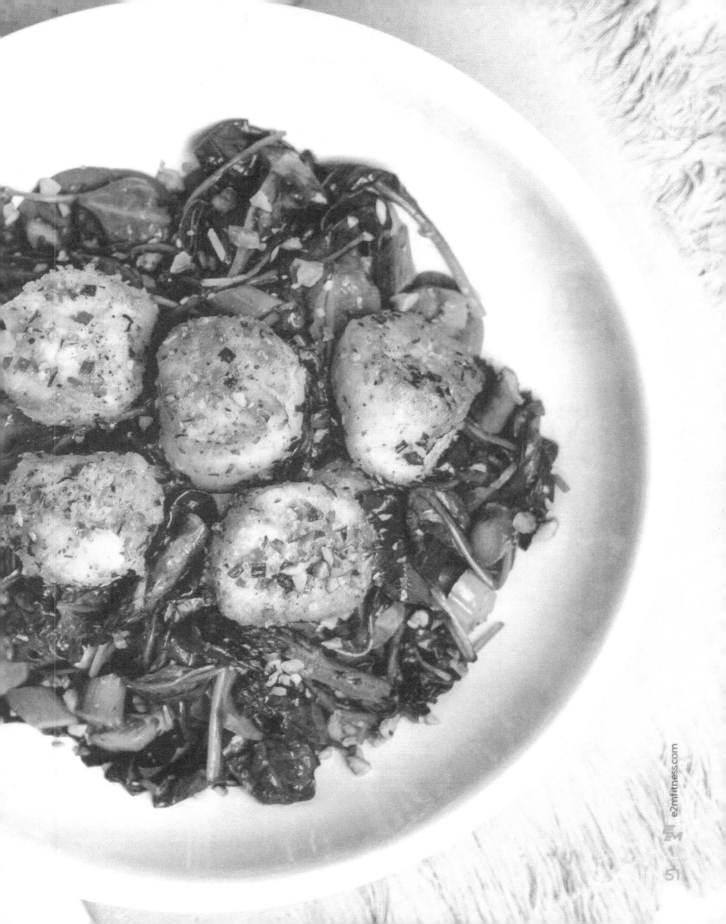

Chili-Lime
Scallops

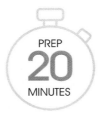

PREP
20
MINUTES

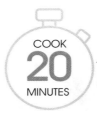

COOK
20
MINUTES

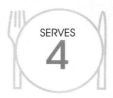

SERVES
4

Ingredients

- *2 pounds sea scallops (20 to 30 per pound)
- 2 tablespoons Chili-Lime seasoning (see page 120)
- Cooking spray
- 1 tablespoon extra-virgin olive oil
- 1 bunch asparagus spears

- 6 cups of spinach
- 1 teaspoon extra-virgin olive oil
- 1 teaspoon sea salt
- ½ teaspoon black pepper
- Lemon zest (for garnish)

Prep

1. For the Chili-Lime Seasoning, whisk together all the ingredients in a small bowl; most of the mixture will be used in this meal.

2. *If using frozen scallops, allow them to thaw overnight in the refrigerator; do not thaw at room temperature. Use paper towels to pat dry the thawed or fresh scallops. Season the scallops on all sides with 1½ tablespoons of the Chili-Lime Seasoning.

Cook

3. Heat a large pan to medium-high heat. When the pan begins to smoke, spray the pan with cooking oil; put the seasoned scallops in the pan. Do not overcrowd the pan, which will cause the scallops to steam; it's best to allow space between and cook in batches. Sauté the scallops until browned, 2 to 3 minutes; flip and cook on the other side until the scallops are slightly firm, 1 to 2 minutes. Remove the scallops from the pan and set aside.

4. Remove the skillet from the heat, and put the spinach in the hot skillet to wilt for 3 to 5 minutes.

5. For the roasted asparagus, first preheat the oven to 400 degrees. Remove the woody part of the spears by snapping off the ends. Discard the ends. Put the trimmed asparagus spears in a shallow bowl or on a platter or baking sheet. Drizzle with 1 tablespoon olive oil, and toss to coat. Season with remaining ½ tablespoon of Chili-Lime Seasoning, sea salt, and black pepper, and toss again.

6. Spray a baking dish with cooking spray. Transfer the asparagus to an oiled baking dish; bake in the preheated oven for 4 to 8 minutes, or until the spears are tender and crisp.

Serve

7. Plate the roasted asparagus and spinach on plates. Top with scallops and garnish with lemon zest.

Lemon-Garlic
Seared Scallops over Zoodles

Ingredients

- *2 pounds sea scallops (20 to 30 per pound)
- ½ teaspoon ground garlic
- ¼ teaspoon sea salt
- ½ teaspoon black pepper
- Cooking spray
- 1 lemon, zested and juiced
- 6 cups zucchini noodles (homemade or store-bought)
- 1 cup thinly sliced mushrooms (baby portabella or cremini)
- 2 tablespoons chopped fresh basil (for garnish)
- Crushed red pepper (optional)

Prep

1. *If using frozen scallops, allow them to thaw overnight in the refrigerator; do not thaw at room temperature. Use paper towels to pat dry the thawed or fresh scallops. Season the scallops on all sides with garlic, sea salt, and black pepper.

Cook

2. Heat a large pan to medium-high heat. When the pan begins to smoke, spray the pan with cooking oil; put the seasoned scallops in the pan. Do not overcrowd the pan, which will cause the scallops to steam; it's best to allow space between and cook in batches. Sauté the scallops until browned, 2 to 3 minutes; flip and cook on the other side until the scallops are slightly firm, 1 to 2 minutes. Remove the scallops from the pan and set aside.

3. Return the pan to medium-high heat and add the juice of ½ lemon in order to deglaze the pan. Add the zucchini noodles and mushrooms. Sauté until the mushrooms are tender, 1 to 2 minutes.

Serve

4. Plate the zoodles and mushrooms, and top with scallops. Garnish with some fresh lemon zest, chopped basil, and the juice from the remaining ½ lemon; sprinkle with optional crushed red pepper.

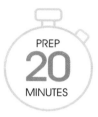

PREP
20
MINUTES

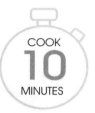

COOK
10
MINUTES

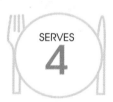

SERVES
4

Note:
Deglazing simply means to add liquid to a hot pan and use a wooden spoon to remove any cooked-on food. This creates a flavorful "sauce" you can cook vegetables in for added flavor.

e2mfitness.com

⁙ Success Stories

Caroline G., Irmo, SC

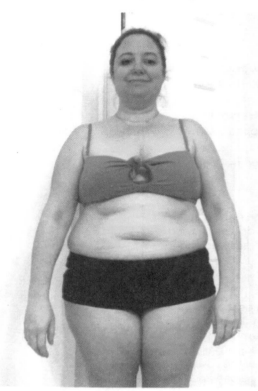
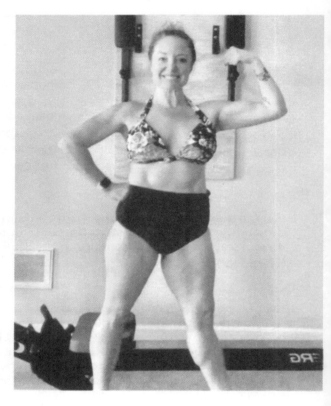

Rounds	Age	Weight Loss
8	41	50

When I found the E2M fitness program, I was extremely overweight, had no energy, had very low self-esteem, and knew I needed to change for the sake of my health and what I could be for my family. Thanks to the simplicity of E2M fitness and the incredibly motivating and supportive community, I've lost fifty pounds, ran a half marathon, and regained my health, my confidence, became a proud example for my teenage daughters, and am a part of a community of like-minded friends.

Non-Scale Victory (NSV)!
Previously, I could not complete running a mile. Recently, I ran 13.1 miles!

Herb Scallops
with Sautéed Spinach and Peppers

Ingredients

Scallops:
- *2 pounds sea scallops (20 to 30 per pound)
- 1 tablespoon Garlic and Herb Seasoning (recipe below)
- Cooking spray

- 1 teaspoon olive oil
- 4 red bell peppers, seeded and thinly sliced
- 8 handfuls spinach

Garlic and Herb Seasoning:
- ¼ tablespoon sea salt
- 1 tablespoon ground garlic
- 1 tablespoon lemon zest
- 2 teaspoons dried rosemary

- 1½ teaspoons dried thyme
- 1½ teaspoons dried oregano
- ¼ teaspoon dried paprika
- ¼ teaspoon crushed red pepper

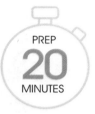

PREP
20
MINUTES

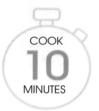

COOK
10
MINUTES

SERVES
4

Prep

1. For the Garlic and Herb Seasoning, whisk together all the ingredients in a small bowl. Transfer to an airtight container or jar.

2. *If using frozen scallops, allow them to thaw overnight in the refrigerator; do not thaw at room temperature. Use paper towels to pat dry the thawed or fresh scallops. Season the scallops on all sides with 1 tablespoon or more if desired of the Garlic and Herb Seasoning.

Cook

3. Heat a large pan to medium-high heat. When the pan begins to smoke, spray the pan with cooking oil; put the seasoned scallops in the pan. Do not overcrowd the pan, which will cause the scallops to steam; it's best to allow space between and cook in batches. Sauté the scallops until browned, 2 to 3 minutes; flip and cook on the other side until the scallops are slightly firm, 1 to 2 minutes. Remove the scallops from the pan and set aside.

4. Add the olive oil to the pan and return to a medium-high heat. Add the sliced red bell peppers and cook for 1 to 2 minutes. Remove the pan from the heat, add the spinach a few handfuls at a time, and mix. Remove the spinach after it begins to wilt, being careful not to overcook it.

Serve

5. Plate the sautéed spinach and peppers, and top with the herb scallops.

≡M Success Stories

Jeneen A., Gastonia, NC

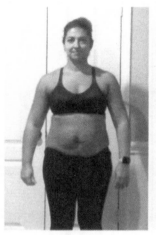 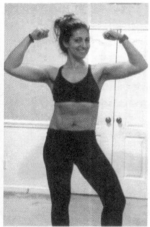

Rounds	Age	Weight Loss
6	42	40

I joined E2M fitness after passing on the opportunity two or three times. I worked out daily and had built up my strength, but I was never ready to commit to a strict meal plan. I ultimately needed to learn what my body needed for fuel. I didn't want to count points, calories, or anything, but just needed my mommy tummy to go.

What is your favorite type of workout?
I love the circuits because they help me continue to get stronger. I never get bored.

Non-Scale Victory (NSV)!
Exposing my stomach in public.

Issac S., Marion, NC

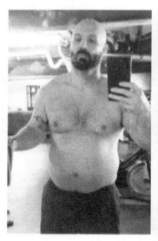 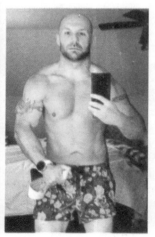

Rounds	Age	Weight Loss
3	37	40

E2M fitness has given me a different outlook on what's important to me. It also has helped me realize that food is fuel and that this lifestyle is sustainable. I'm never starving or miserable.

What is your favorite type of workout?
I like upper body HIITs and full bodies with Brad. It feels like his messages are talking directly to me and they help push me every week to be better.

What does the E2M community mean to you?
It means everything. I have more energy. I feel better, look better, sleep better, and I enjoy life much more.

Low-Carb Banh Mi
Scallop Bowl

Ingredients

- *2 pounds sea scallops (20 to 30 per pound)
- 1 tablespoon ground garlic
- ½ teaspoon ground ginger
- ¼ teaspoon sea salt
- ⅛ teaspoon black pepper
- Cooking spray
- 2 limes fresh, juice and zest

- 2 cups shredded purple cabbage
- 4 cups riced cauliflower (frozen or shelf stable)
- 1 cup chopped cilantro, divided
- 1 cup shredded carrots
- 1 cup thinly sliced cucumbers
- 1 jalapeño, seeded and thinly sliced (optional)

Prep

1. *If using frozen scallops, allow them to thaw overnight in the refrigerator; do not thaw at room temperature. Use paper towels to pat dry the thawed or fresh scallops. Season the scallops on all sides with the garlic, ginger, sea salt, and black pepper.

Cook

2. Heat a large pan to medium-high heat. When the pan begins to smoke, spray the pan with cooking oil; put the seasoned scallops in the pan. Do not overcrowd the pan, which will cause the scallops to steam; it's best to allow space between and cook in batches. Sauté the scallops until browned, 2 to 3 minutes; flip and cook on the other side until the scallops are slightly firm, 1 to 2 minutes. Remove the scallops from the pan and set aside.

3. Return the pan to medium-high heat, and add the juice of one lime to deglaze the pan. Add the shredded purple cabbage and sauté for 3-5 minutes, until slightly softened. Remove from the pan and set aside. Add the riced cauliflower to the pan and sauté for 3 to 5 minutes. Add half of the chopped cilantro and the remaining fresh lime juice. Toss to combine.

Serve

4. Divide the riced cauliflower and purple cabbage between the bowls. Top with the shredded carrots, sliced cucumbers, and scallops. Garnish with fresh jalapeño slices and the remaining chopped cilantro and lime zest.

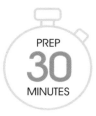

PREP
30
MINUTES

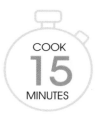

COOK
15
MINUTES

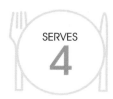

SERVES
4

Note:

Deglazing simply means to add liquid to a hot pan and use a wooden spoon to remove any cooked-on food. This creates a flavorful "sauce" you can cook vegetables in for added flavor.

Banh mi is a traditional Vietnamese sandwich made with pork, carrots, cucumber, cilantro, and red chili pepper. This low-carb version has all the same powerful flavors you can enjoy on plan!

e2mfitness.com

Seared Scallops
with Avocado-Cucumber Salad

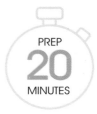

PREP
20
MINUTES

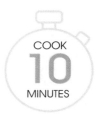

COOK
10
MINUTES

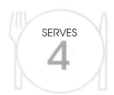

SERVES
4

Ingredients

Avocado-Cucumber Salad:

- 2 English cucumbers, thinly sliced
- 2 avocados, peeled and diced
- 1 lemon, zested and juiced
- 1 teaspoon dried dill
- ¼ teaspoon sea salt
- ½ teaspoon black pepper
- 6 handfuls of spring mix

Scallops:

- *2 pounds sea scallops (20 to 30 per pound)
- Cooking spray
- 2 tablespoons Chili-Lime Seasoning (see page 120)

Prep

1. For the Chili-Lime Seasoning, whisk together all the ingredients in a small bowl; most of the mixture will be used in this meal.

2. Prepare the avocado-cucumber salad by combining the sliced cucumber, diced avocado, lemon zest, lemon juice, dill, sea salt, and black pepper. Set aside until ready to serve.

3. *If using frozen scallops, allow them to thaw overnight in the refrigerator; do not thaw at room temperature. Use paper towels to pat dry the thawed or fresh scallops. Season the scallops on all sides with 1½ tablespoons of the Chili-Lime Seasoning.

Cook

4. Heat a large pan to medium-high heat. When the pan begins to smoke, spray the pan with cooking oil; put the seasoned scallops in the pan. Do not overcrowd the pan, which will cause the scallops to steam; it's best to allow space between and cook in batches. Sauté the scallops until browned, 2 to 3 minutes; flip and cook on the other side until the scallops are slightly firm, 1 to 2 minutes.

Serve

5. Plate spring mix. Divide the avocado-cucumber salad between the plates, and top with the seared scallops.

Note:
This dish pairs well with the Avocado Lime Dressing (see page 115)

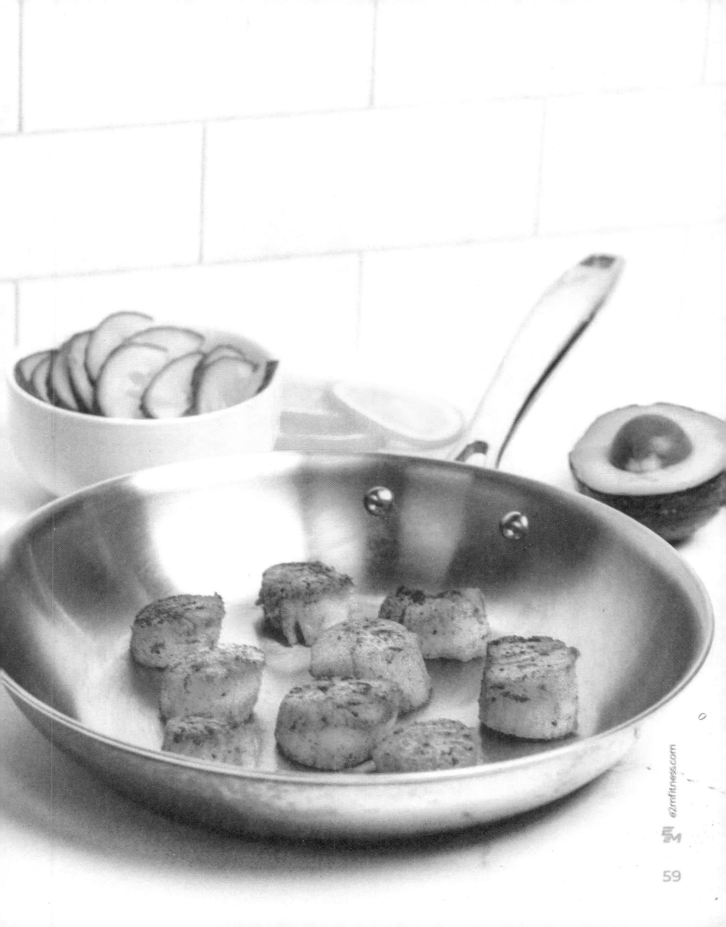

Matthew and Jessica H., Lincolnton, NC

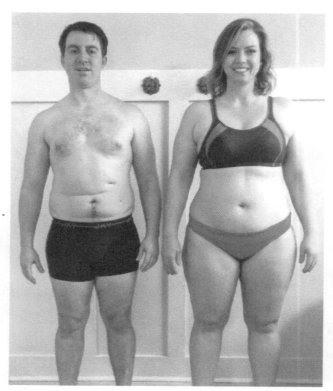 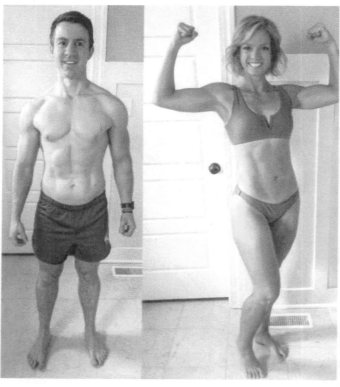

Rounds	Age	combined Weight Loss
4	38	100

We were high school sweethearts who dated through college, got married, worked full time, had two children, and lost focus on ourselves and our health. We joined the E2M program in our worst physical condition, not knowing two weeks later COVID-19 would shut down the world. Instead of focusing on the negatives of COVID and continuing to decline in physical fitness, E2M fitness provided the structure we needed to excel physically and mentally during the pandemic. Thanks to our E2M fitness journey, our relationship is the closest it's ever been, we're in the best shape of our lives by a long shot, we've reconnected with old friends, we've gained new friends, and we've built the discipline to live this sustainable lifestyle!

What is your favorite type of workout?
The ones that leave you drenched, on the floor, and gasping for air.

Non-Scale Victory (NSV)!
We purposely plan beach vacations to enjoy our E2M fitness results.

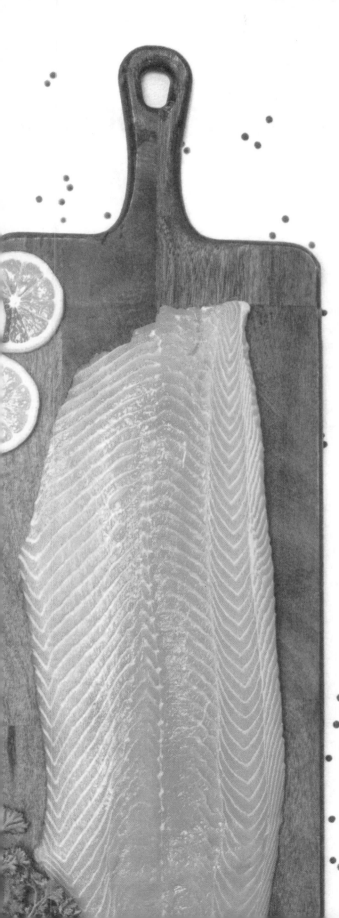

Whole Fish

Chia Seed Salmon
with Roasted Asparagus

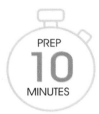

PREP
10
MINUTES

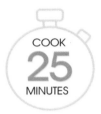

COOK
25
MINUTES

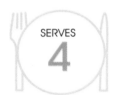

SERVES
4

Ingredients

Salmon:
- 4 (4 to 6 ounces each) salmon fillets
- 2 tablespoons mustard
- ½ teaspoon ground garlic
- ½ teaspoon dried parsley
- ½ teaspoon thyme
- ½ teaspoon sea salt
- ½ teaspoon black pepper
- 2 tablespoons chia seeds
- Cooking spray

Asparagus:
- 2 bunches asparagus
- 2 tablespoons extra-virgin olive oil
- 1 tablespoon sea salt
- ½ tablespoon black pepper

Prep

1. Preheat the oven to 400 degrees. Line a baking sheet with parchment paper or spray with cooking oil.

2. To prepare the salmon, first mix the mustard, garlic, parsley, thyme, sea salt, and black pepper in a bowl. Brush each salmon fillet with about ½ tablespoon of the mustard mixture. Sprinkle ½ tablespoon of the chia seeds on top of each fillet. Set aside on the lined baking sheet.

3. To prepare the asparagus, remove the woody part of the spears by snapping off the ends. Discard the ends. Put the trimmed asparagus spears in a bowl. Drizzle with the olive oil, and toss with your hands to evenly coat. Season with sea salt and black pepper, and toss again.

4. Preheat the grill to medium heat, about 375 degrees.

Cook

5. To cook the salmon, heat a large pan over medium-high heat, spray with cooking oil; sear the salmon for 1 minute just on the top side. Transfer from the pan back to the lined baking sheet. Bake at 400 degrees for 15 minutes, or until the salmon reaches an internal temperature of 145 degrees.

6. While the salmon is in the oven, cook the asparagus. Lay the spears across the grill grates or indoor grill pan, perpendicular to the bars. Grill for 4 to 8 minutes with the lid closed, or until the spears are tender and crisp. Half through cooking, use tongs to roll the spears for even grill marks.

Serve

7. Plate the asparagus and top with a serving of salmon.

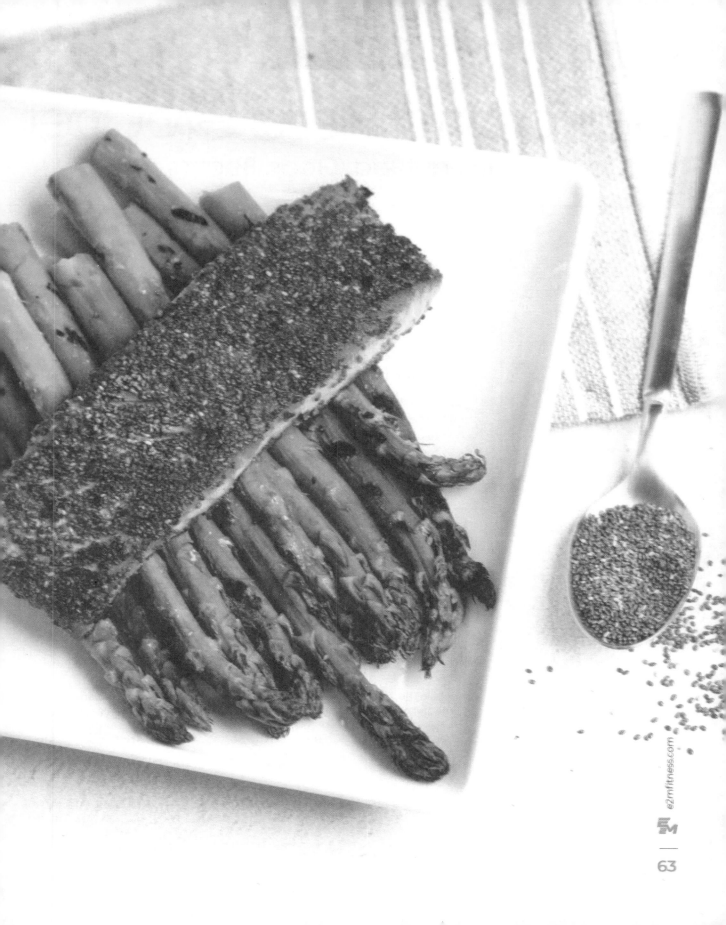

Garlic and Herb Grouper
with Sautéed Green Beanss

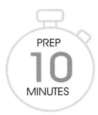

PREP
10
MINUTES

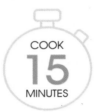

COOK
15
MINUTES

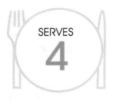

SERVES
4

Ingredients

Fish:
- 4 (4 to 6 ounces each) fresh grouper or any white fish, skin removed
- 1 tablespoon ground garlic
- 1 teaspoon sea salt
- ½ teaspoon black pepper
- 1 teaspoon dried thyme
- 1 teaspoon dried parsley
- 1 lemon (for zest)
- Cooking spray

Green Beans:
- 1 tablespoon olive oil
- ¼ teaspoon crushed red pepper
- ½ teaspoon ground garlic
- 2 pounds green beans, ends trimmed
- 1 teaspoon sea salt
- 1 teaspoon fresh thyme (or ¼ teaspoon dried thyme)
- ¼ teaspoon black pepper
- 1 cup drained and diced black olives

Prep

1. Preheat the oven to 350 degrees. Line a baking sheet with parchment paper or spray with cooking oil.

2. To prepare the fish, combine the garlic, sea salt, black pepper, thyme, and parsley; season the fish on both sides with the spice mixture. Put the fish on the baking sheet and zest the lemon over the top of the fish.

Cook

3. Bake the fish for 8 minutes, or until it reaches an internal temperature of 145 degrees.

4. While the fish is in the oven, make the green beans. In a large pan over medium heat, heat the olive oil, crushed red pepper, and garlic just until sizzling, then add the green beans; sauté for 4 to 5 minutes, until the green beans are cooked. Add the fresh thyme, sea salt, and black pepper; toss to mix well.

Serve

5. Plate the green beans, top with the fish, and add black olives to each serving.

Lemon Dill Halibut
with Roasted Brussels Sprouts

Ingredients

Fish:
- Cooking spray
- 2 pounds halibut or other white flaky fish
- 1 tablespoon dried dill
- 1 teaspoon sea salt
- ½ teaspoon dried smoked paprika
- ½ teaspoon ground garlic
- 1 lemon, zested and juiced

Brussels Sprouts:
- 8 cups brussels sprouts, quartered
- 3 tablespoons spicy brown mustard
- 3 tablespoons olive oil or avocado oil
- ½ tablespoon ground garlic
- ½ tablespoon dried paprika
- ½ tablespoon sea salt
- 1 teaspoon black pepper

Olive Tapenade Topping:
- 1 can (6 ounces) black olives, drained and diced
- 1 tablespoon dried dill
- 1 tablespoon ground garlic
- ½ lemon, zested and juiced

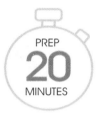

PREP
20
MINUTES

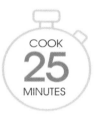

COOK
25
MINUTES

SERVES
4

Prep

1. Preheat the oven to 400 degrees.

2. Line a sheet pan with parchment paper or spray with cooking oil. Spray cooking oil on the fish; season with the salt, dill, paprika, garlic, lemon zest, and lemon juice.

3. To make the brussels sprouts, cut in half to ensure they cook evenly. Put the pieces in a large bowl and add the spicy brown mustard, olive oil, garlic, and paprika; toss together.

Cook

4. Bake the fish at 400 degrees for 15 to 20 minutes, or until it reaches an internal temperature of 145 degrees. You can bake the brussels sprouts at the same time, but they will need to cook a little longer than the fish.

5. For the brussels sprouts, either roast in a cast-iron skillet or greased baking dish at 400 degrees for a total of 20-25 minutes. **Air fryer option:** Cook at 400 degrees for 15 minutes.

6. For the olive tapenade topping, combine the diced olives, dill, garlic, and the juice and zest of ½ lemon.

Serve

7. Plate the roasted brussels sprouts; top each serving with a halibut fillet and olive tapenade.

e2mfitness.com

Seared Ahi Tuna
Bowl

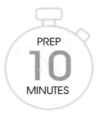

**PREP
10
MINUTES**

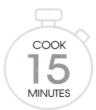

**COOK
15
MINUTES**

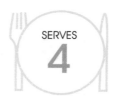

**SERVES
4**

Ingredients

- 4 sashimi-grade tuna steaks
- 2 tablespoons avocado oil
- 2 tablespoons sesame seeds
- 1½ teaspoons dried paprika
- 1½ teaspoons ground garlic
- ¼ teaspoon sea salt
- ⅛ teaspoon black pepper
- 1 lime, juice

- 8 cups fresh or frozen cauliflower rice
- 1 cucumber, thinly sliced
- ½ red onion, sliced thin
- 1 jalapeño, sliced thin
- Cilantro Lime Dressing (see page 113)
- Cooking spray

Prep

1. Pat dry the tuna steaks with paper towels. Rub avocado oil on both sides of the steaks. Combine the sesame seeds, paprika, garlic, sea salt, and black pepper on a plate. Press the tuna steaks into the spice blend until every side is completely covered.

Cook

2. In an oiled, hot pan, sear each side for 30 seconds to 1 minute for rare tuna steaks. Sear longer if preferred. Remove from pan. Add the juice of 1/2 lime to pan to deglaze. Add in cauliflower rice and sauté for 3-5 min.

3. Combine the cauliflower rice, with 2 tablespoon of Cilantro Lime Dressing and mix to combine.

Serve

4. Plate cauliflower rice, top with seared tuna steak, red onion, cucumber and jalapenos. Finish with squeeze of fresh lime.

Note:

This beautiful finished dish looks intimidating, but it preps and cooks quickly. The most important ingredient is the sushi-grade tuna; ask your fishmonger for the appropriate variety.

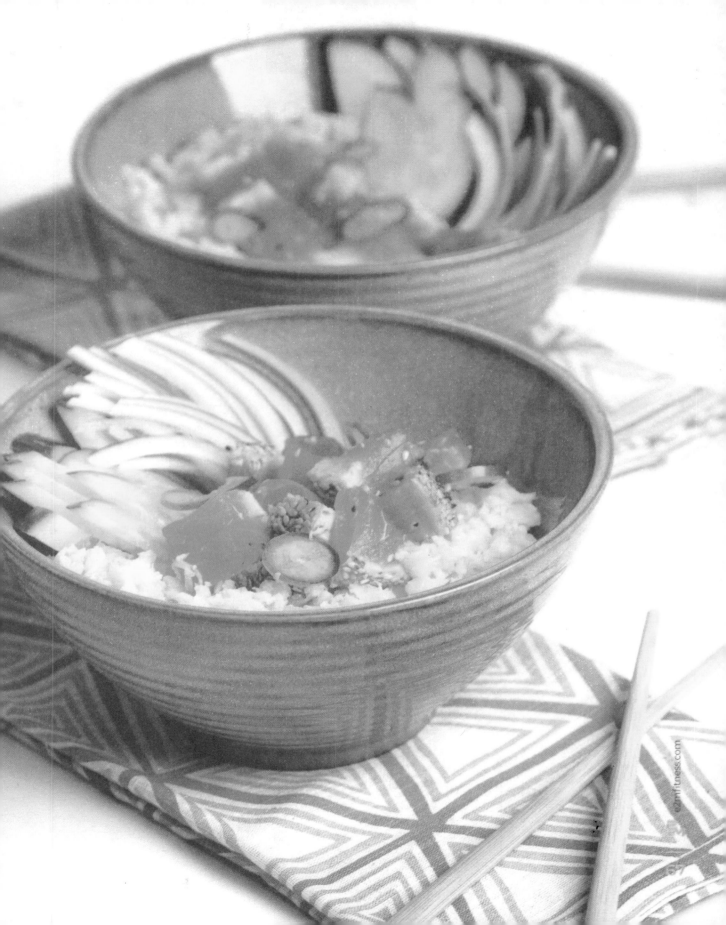

Ahi Tuna Steaks
with Cilantro Slaw

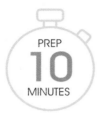

PREP
10
MINUTES

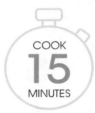

COOK
15
MINUTES

SERVES
4

Ingredients

Tuna:
- 6 oz sashimi-grade tuna steaks
- 2 tablespoons avocado or olive oil
- 1 tablespoon sesame seeds
- 1 tablespoon ground garlic
- 1 tablespoon dried paprika
- 1 teaspoon ground ginger
- ½ teaspoon sea salt
- ⅛ teaspoon black pepper
- Cooking spray

Cilantro Slaw
- 5 cups shredded cabbage
- 2 cups shredded carrots
- 1 cucumber, thinly sliced
- 1 tablespoon avocado oil
- 2 tablespoons rice wine vinegar
- ½ cup fresh chopped cilantro, divided
- 1 teaspoon sea salt
- 1 lime, juice and zest

Prep

1. Pat dry the tuna steaks with paper towels. Rub avocado or olive oil on both sides. Combine the sesame seeds, garlic, paprika, ginger, sea salt, and black pepper on a plate. Press the tuna steaks into the dry rub, covering all sides.

Cook

2. In an oiled, hot pan, sear each side for 30 seconds to 1 minute for rare tuna steaks. Sear longer if preferred.

3. Combine the shredded cabbage, shredded carrots, and sliced cucumbers in a bowl. Add the avocado oil, rice wine vinegar, lime juice, zest, ¼ cup chopped cilantro, and salt. Toss to combine.

Serve

4. Arrange the cilantro slaw on plates and top with tuna. Garnish with the remaining fresh cilantro.

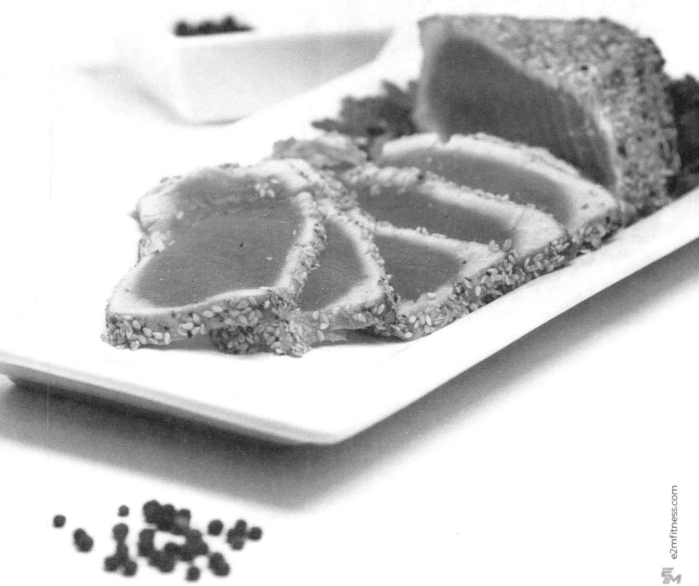

Dawn B., Lebanon, CT

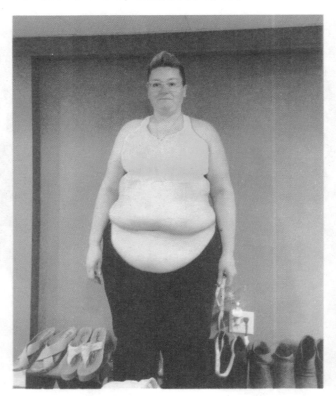 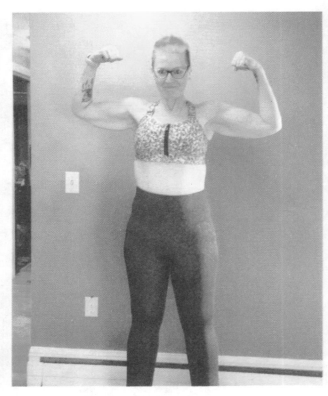

Rounds	Age	Weight Loss
8	38	141

I am a cancer survivor. I have lymphedema. I had never worked out a day in my life. I ate whatever I wanted. I was a proud "I love me and my curves" girl. The swelling in my legs and cellulitis caused me to be in pain all the time. Then I found E2M fitness and my life changed in every single way—one hundred and forty-one pounds gone forever! That's a whole dang human! I could have never done it without the support of all of you!

What does the E2M community mean to you?
The E2M community has completely changed my life inside and out.

Non-Scale Victory (NSV)!
My lymphedema is finally under control.

Spicy Jerk Salmon
with Sautéed Green Beans and Peppers

Ingredients

Salmon:

- 4 (4 to 6 ounces each) salmon fillets
- Cooking spray
- 2 tablespoons Jerk Seasoning (see page 121)

Vegetables:

- 2 tablespoons extra-virgin olive oil
- ¼ teaspoon crushed red pepper
- ½ teaspoon ground garlic
- 2 pound green beans, ends trimmed
- 1 red bell pepper, seeded and thinly sliced
- 1 yellow bell pepper, seeded and thinly sliced
- 1 can black olives, drained, sliced
- 1 teaspoon fresh thyme (or ¼ teaspoon dried thyme)
- 1 teaspoon sea salt
- ¼ teaspoon black pepper

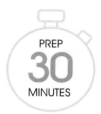

PREP
30
MINUTES

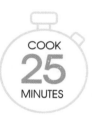

COOK
25
MINUTES

SERVES
4

Prep

1. Preheat the oven to 400 degrees.

2. Whisk together all the Jerk Seasoning ingredients in a small bowl. Transfer to an airtight container or jar.

3. Evenly distribute the jerk seasoning over each of the salmon fillets. Line a sheet pan with parchment paper or spray with cooking spray.

Cook

4. Heat a large pan on medium-high heat; spray with cooking oil and sear the salmon for 1 minute just on the top side. Once finished, transfer it to the sheet pan. Bake for 15 to 20 minutes, or until the salmon reaches an internal temperature of 145 degrees.

5. While the salmon is baking, make the green beans. Heat the olive oil in a large wide-bottomed pan. Add the crushed red pepper and garlic; cook just until sizzling, then add the trimmed green beans, sliced red bell pepper, sliced yellow bell pepper, and olives. Cook for 4 to 5 minutes, until the beans are cooked and flavored with the oil mixture. Add the thyme, sea salt, and black pepper. Toss to mix well.

Serve

6. Plate the green beans and peppers and top with salmon.

Mediterranean Cod
and Vegetables

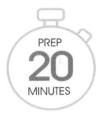

PREP
20
MINUTES

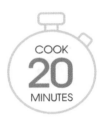

COOK
20
MINUTES

SERVES
4

Ingredients

Fish:
- 4 (6 ounces each) halibut or cod fillets
- 1 lemon (juice and zest for garnish)
- ½ of the Mediterranean Blend recipe

Vegetable Marinade:
- 1½ tablespoons olive oil
- 1 tablespoon red wine vinegar
- 1 medium bunch asparagus, chopped
- 1 can (14 ounces) artichoke hearts, drained, chopped
- 1 jar (12 ounces) roasted red peppers, drained, chopped
- 1 can (6 ounces) black olives, drained, sliced
- 2 tablespoons of the Mediterranean Blend recipe (see page 120)

Prep

1. Combine all the Mediterranean Blend ingredients; all of the blend will be used in this meal.

2. Preheat the oven to 400 degrees.

3. To prepare the vegetable marinade, combine the olive oil, red wine vinegar, asparagus, artichoke hearts, roasted red peppers, and olives in a large bowl. Sprinkle 1 tablespoon of the prepared seasoning blend over the mixture. Cover and refrigerate for 30 minutes.

4. While the vegetables are marinating, line a sheet pan with parchment paper or cooking spray. Put the fish on the pan and season both sides of the fillets with the remaining prepared seasoning blend.

Cook

5. Roast at 400 degrees for 15 to 20 minutes, or until the fish reaches an internal temperature of 145 degrees. Optional: broil 2 to 3 minutes, or until the fillets brown on top.

Serve:

6. Divide and arrange the cold marinated vegetables on plates. Top with a serving of fish and garnish with fresh lemon juice and zest.

Meal prep idea:
Prepare the fish and vegetables. Let the fish cool, and store in an airtight container; store the vegetables separately. Keep in the refrigerator for up to three days.

Seared Citrus Tuna
with Bok Choy

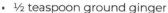

Ingredients

Seared Tuna:

- 4 sushi-grade ahi tuna steaks
- ¼ cup black sesame seeds
- ½ cup white sesame seeds
- ½ teaspoon sea salt
- ½ teaspoon black pepper

- 1 orange (for zest)
- 1 lemon (for zest)
- 2 tablespoons olive oil
- 4 (6 ounces each) tuna steaks, 1-inch thick

Bok Choy:

- 2 heads bok choy, sliced, both white and green parts
- 1 teaspoon olive oil
- 1½ teaspoons sesame seeds
- ½ teaspoon ground garlic

- ½ teaspoon ground ginger
- ½ teaspoon crushed red pepper
- ½ teaspoon sea salt
- ½ teaspoon black pepper

Prep

1. In a shallow dish or plate, combine the black sesame seeds, white sesame seeds, sea salt, black pepper, orange zest, and lemon zest; stir to mix. Pat dry the tuna steaks with paper towels. Rub the olive oil on the tuna steaks; press the tuna steaks into the sesame seed mixture, coating the tuna evenly on all sides.

Cook

2. Rinse the bok choy. Heat the olive oil in a large sauté pan over medium heat. Add the garlic, ginger, and crushed red pepper; heat until fragrant, 2 to 3 minutes. Add the bok choy and sauté for about 8 minutes. You may need to cook in batches to not overcrowd the pan. Season with sea salt and black pepper.

3. In a large pan over medium heat, warm the olive oil until smoking; arrange the tuna in the pan (making sure not to overcrowd), and cook until the white sesame seeds start to turn golden underneath (about 1 minute). Carefully turn the tuna over and cook for about another minute. Transfer the tuna to a cutting board and let rest. Cut into ¼-inch-thick slices.

Serve

4. Plate the bok choy and top with sliced tuna. Sprinkle each plate with the remaining sesame seeds.

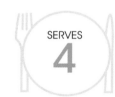

PREP
15
MINUTES

COOK
15
MINUTES

SERVES
4

e2mfitness.com

E2M Success Stories

Crystal D., Spartanburg, SC

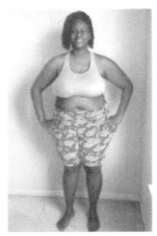 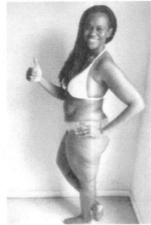

Rounds	Age	Weight Loss
13	40	75

I wanted to get healthier and stronger to become a better model of health for my children. I was the girl who knew all the right things I needed to do to lose weight, but struggled with putting all of those components together! The E2M program showed me the way!

What does the E2M community mean to you?
The E2M community was the biggest determining factor for me to have successfully completed my first eight-week round!

Non-Scale Victory (NSV)!
I can comfortably sit within restaurant booths.

Kate R., Lancashire, U.K.

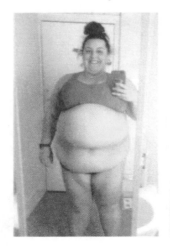 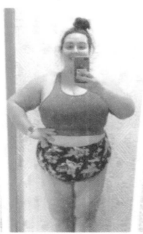

Rounds	Age	Weight Loss
3	36	70

The E2M fitness program has changed my life. The support and accountability I get from the group and the team are unrivaled! I've achieved things I thought were impossible and it's all because of this magnificent program!

What does the E2M community mean to you?
It means everything to me! There is nowhere like it on the internet. From the other side of the world, I've made my best friends through this group!

Non-Scale Victory (NSV)!
No more seatbelt extenders for me and I can now climb mountains!

Cajun Salmon
with Garlic Roasted Okra

Ingredients

Fish:

- 4 (4 to 6 ounces each) salmon fillets, skin on or off
- Cooking spray
- 1 teaspoon sea salt
- 2 tablespoons Cajun Blend (see page 123)
- 1 tablespoon olive oil
- 1 tablespoon lemon juice

Okra:

- 2 pounds okra
- 1½ teaspoons dried paprika
- 1½ teaspoons ground garlic
- ½ teaspoon sea salt
- 1½ tablespoons olive oil

Prep

1. For the Cajun Blend, whisk together all the ingredients in a small bowl. Transfer to an airtight container or jar.

2. To prepare the salmon, pat dry the salmon with paper towels. Generously spray the fillets with cooking spray, then sprinkle the fillets with the sea salt and Cajun Seasoning.

3. Preheat oven to 400 degrees. Line a baking sheet with parchment paper or spray with cooking oil.

4. To prepare the okra, rinse the okra and dry with a paper towel. Trim the stem ends, then cut the okra in half length wise. Put the okra into a medium-size mixing bowl. In a small dish, mix the paprika, garlic, and sea salt. Sprinkle the seasoning mix over the okra and add the olive oil. Mix until well coated; spread out the okra evenly on the baking sheet.

Cook

5. Bake the okra for about 15 minutes while cooking the salmon.

6. To cook the salmon, first heat the olive oil in a large skillet over medium-high heat. Add the salmon, skin side up, and sear for 2 to 3 minutes, until cooked about halfway to the center of thickest part of fillet. Flip the salmon with a fish spatula. Drizzle with the lemon juice, and spoon the pan juices over the salmon. Cook for another 2 to 5 minutes, depending on the thickness, until just tender or the salmon reaches an internal temperature of 145 degrees.

Serve

7. Plate the roasted okra and salmon.

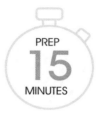

PREP
15
MINUTES

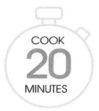

COOK
20
MINUTES

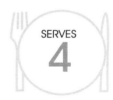

SERVES
4

Dijon Salmon
with Spinach-Avocado Salad

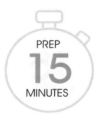

PREP
15
MINUTES

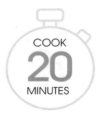

COOK
20
MINUTES

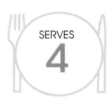

SERVES
4

Ingredients

- 4 (6 ounces each) salmon fillets
- 2 tablespoons Dijon mustard
- 2 avocados, peeled and diced
- 6 cups chopped spinach
- 1½ teaspoons olive oil
- 2 red peppers, seeded and thinly sliced
- 1 tablespoon Everything Seasoning (see page 125)
- 1 lemon, zested and juiced

Prep

1. Preheat the oven to 400 degrees. Line a sheet pan with parchment paper or spray with cooking spray, and put the salmon fillets on the pan. Spoon a ½ tablespoon of the Dijon mustard onto each salmon fillet; spread evenly. (Prepare the salad once the salmon is in the oven.)

Cook

2. Bake the salmon for 15 to 20 minutes, or until the salmon reaches an internal temperature of 145 degrees.

3. While the salmon is in the oven, prepare the salad. In a large bowl, combine the diced avocados, chopped spinach, and red peppers. Add the olive oil, Everything Seasoning, and lemon juice and zest. Toss to mix well.

Serve

4. Divide the spinach-avocado salad on plates and top with salmon.

Roasted Chili-Lime
Salmon with Kale

Ingredients

Salmon:

- 1½ teaspoons chili powder
- 1 teaspoon ground cumin
- 1 teaspoon ground garlic
- 1 teaspoon onion powder
- 1 teaspoon ground coriander
- 1 teaspoon sea salt
- ¼ teaspoon ground cayenne pepper
- 1 tablespoon oil
- 1 lime, zested and juiced
- 4 (6 ounces each) salmon fillets
- Cooking spray

Kale:

- 4 medium bunches Tuscan kale, or bagged kale greens (about 24 ounces)
- 2 tablespoons olive oil
- ½ teaspoon ground garlic
- 1 teaspoon sea salt
- ½ teaspoon black pepper
- 2 avocados, peeled and diced
- 1 lime, zest and juice

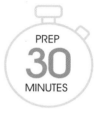

PREP
30
MINUTES

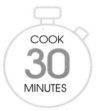

COOK
30
MINUTES

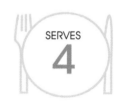

SERVES
4

Prep

1. Combine the chili powder, cumin, garlic, onion powder, coriander, sea salt, and cayenne pepper. Set aside. Combine the oil, lime zest and juice, and the combined spice blend. Mix everything together. Spoon the mixture onto the salmon fillets and coat evenly; refrigerate for 30 minutes to marinate.

2. Preheat the oven to 400 degrees so that the oven is almost ready when the salmon is finished marinating.

3. Line a baking sheet with parchment paper or spray cooking oil and put the salmon on top. (Prepare the kale once the salmon is in the oven.)

Cook

4. Bake the salmon for 15 to 20 minutes, or until the salmon reaches an internal temperature of 145 degrees. Increase the oven temperature to 425 degrees once the salmon is done.

5. To prepare the kale, first line a baking sheet with parchment paper. Chop the kale. In a large bowl, mix the kale with the olive oil, garlic, sea salt, and black pepper. Spread the kale leaves on the baking sheet in a single layer.

6. Roast the kale for 5 minutes at 425 degrees. Remove the pan, stir, and roast another 2 minutes. Remove the pan from the oven one more time, stir, and roast 2 minutes more or until the kale is wilted and crispy on the edges.

Serve

7. Plate the roasted kale and salmon; top with diced avocado. Finish with fresh lime juice and zest.

Mahi Fish Tacos
with Citrus Cabbage Slaw

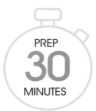

PREP
30
MINUTES

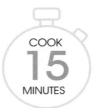

COOK
15
MINUTES

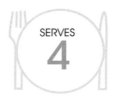

SERVES
4

Ingredients

Fish:
- 2 pounds mahi-mahi or your favorite fish
- 2 tablespoons Asian Spice Blend
- 1 tablespoon olive oil
- Cooking spray
- 1 head butter lettuce, leaves rinsed and separated
- 1 cup peanuts, crushed (optional for garnish)
- ¼ cup cilantro, chopped (optional for garnish)

Citrus Cabbage Slaw:
- 1 Thai chili pepper, thinly sliced (omit if you prefer no spice)
- 1 tablespoon Asian Spice Blend (see page 125)
- 4 cups thinly shredded cabbage slaw mix, or 1 bag packaged
- ¼ teaspoon sea salt
- ⅛ teaspoon black pepper
- 1 lime, zested and juiced
- 1 orange, zested and juiced

Prep

1. For the Asian Spice Blend, whisk together all the ingredients in a small bowl. Transfer to an airtight container or jar.

2. To prepare the fish, cut the fish into approximately ½-inch cubes, and put into a mixing bowl. Add 2 tablespoons of the Asian Spice Blend and the olive oil, and mix well; refrigerate for 20 minutes.

3. Preheat the oven to 375 degrees. Line a baking sheet with parchment paper or with cooking spray.

4. To make the citrus cabbage slaw, combine the lime zest and juice, orange zest and juice, sliced Thai chili (if using), and 1 tablespoon of the Asian Spice Blend with the cabbage slaw mix; marinate in the refrigerator for at least 30 minutes.

Cook

5. Evenly spread the fish on the pan. Bake for 4 to 6 minutes, or until the fish reaches an internal temperature of 145 degrees. You may need to cook i batches to not overcrowd the pan.

Serve

6. Plate the lettuce leaves and top with slaw and cooked fish; garnish with optional crushed peanuts and chopped cilantro, if desired.

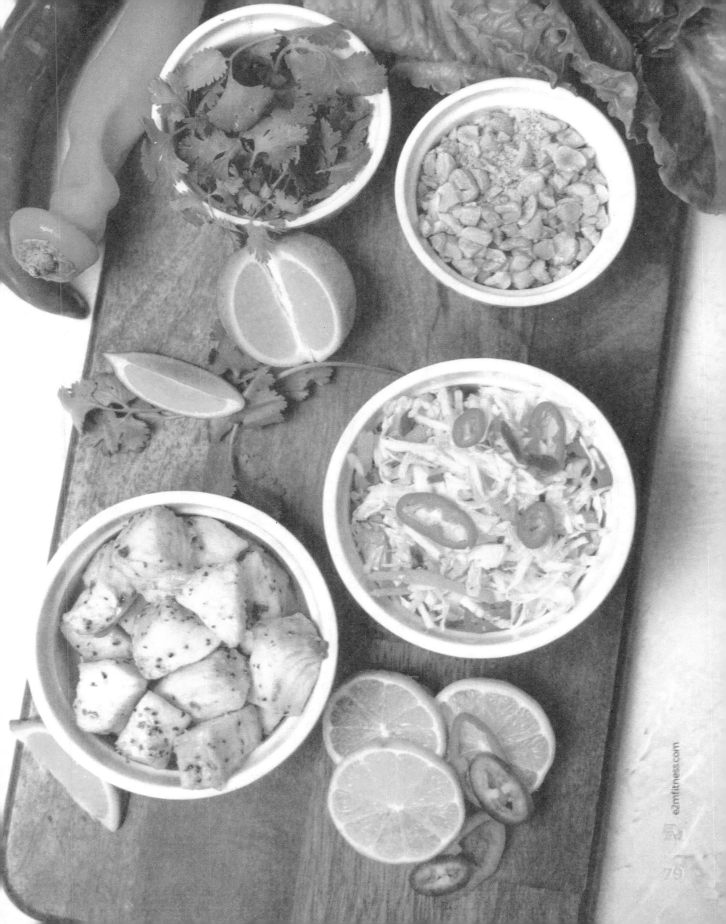

Barrett N., Lexington, SC

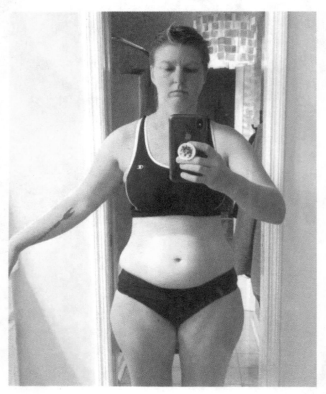 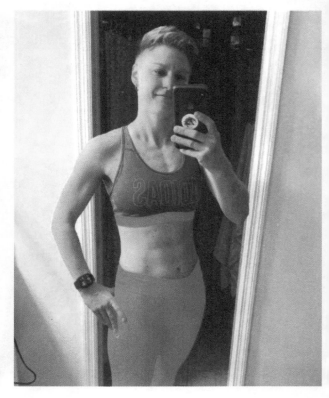

Rounds	Age	Weight Loss
2	**39**	**37**

What were you hoping to gain from your E2M experience?
I was hoping to gain a more fit body (and I did), but what I really gained was confidence, the most amazing friends and girlfriend, and discipline. I'm forever grateful to Jeff for creating—and all the coaches for implementing—the most wonderful life-changing fitness program on the planet for your mind, body, and soul!

Non-Scale Victory (NSV)!
Gaining confidence in who I am and feeling better than I ever have, led me to meet the love of my life within the E2M fitness program.

Lemon Pepper
Sheet-Pan Salmon and Collard Greens

Ingredients

Collard Greens:

- 1 large bunch collard greens or large bag chopped collard greens
- 2 tablespoons dried smoked paprika
- 1 tablespoon minced garlic
- 2 tablespoons ground mustard
- 1½ teaspoons black pepper
- 4 cups of water or enough to cover
- 2 tablespoons olive or avocado oil

Salmon Marinade:

- 4 (6 ounces each) salmon fillets
- 1 tablespoon rice vinegar
- 1 tablespoon olive oil
- 1 lemon, zested and juiced
- 1½ teaspoons sesame seeds
- ½ teaspoon minced garlic
- ¼ teaspoon black pepper
- 2 avocados, peeled, sliced
- 2 tablespoons Lemon Pepper Seasoning (see page 120)

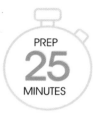

PREP
25
MINUTES

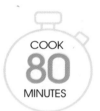

COOK
80
MINUTES

SERVES
4

Prep

1. To prepare the collard greens, rinse thoroughly, as collard greens tend to be very dirty and contain dirt and sand. If you're not using store-bought chopped collard greens, slice the collard green leaves down the center and remove the stem. Stack the leaves and roll, slicing the collards leaves into strips.

2. Add 2 tablespoons of oil to a dutch oven or deep-sided pot. Add the paprika, garlic, ground mustard, and black pepper to the pot and allow the spices to heat; add in the collard greens and stir to mix with the spices. Pour in the water and bring to a boil for 20 minutes; turn down the heat and allow to simmer for at least 1 hour.

3. In a large bowl, whisk together the rice vinegar, olive oil, lemon zest, lemon juice, sesame seeds, garlic, and black pepper. Add the salmon fillets one at a time, coating each with the marinade. Cover a large sheet pan with parchment paper or cooking spray. Put the salmon fillets on the sheet pan, skin side down.

4. Refrigerate and let marinate for 20 minutes.

5. Preheat the oven to 400 degrees.

Cook

6. Bake the salmon for 15 to 20 minutes, or until the salmon reaches an internal temperature of 145 degrees.

Serve

7. Plate the collard greens and diced avocado; top with salmon and finish with the juice of ½ lemon.

Note:
If your family loves salmon and traditional southern collard greens, this is a wonderful healthy twist for your weeknight dinners!

e2mfitness.com

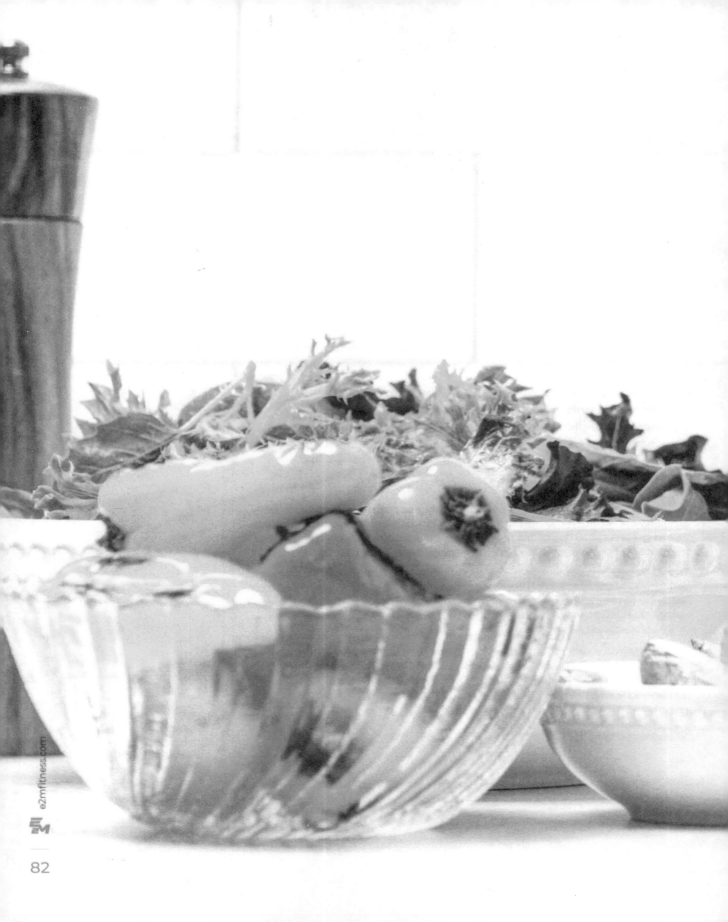

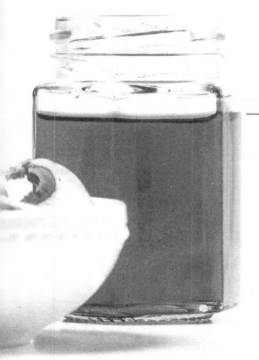

Salads

Herb Roasted
Salmon Salad

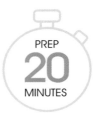

PREP
20
MINUTES

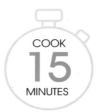

COOK
15
MINUTES

SERVES
4

Ingredients

Salmon:
- 1 teaspoon dried rosemary
- 1 teaspoon dried thyme
- 1 teaspoon fresh chives , snipped
- 1 teaspoon sea salt
- ¼ teaspoon black pepper
- 4 (6 ounces each) salmon fillets, skin removed
- 2 tablespoons Dijon mustard
- Cooking spray
- 1½ cups sliced button mushrooms

Salad Base:
- 4 cups baby kale
- 4 cups broccoli slaw
- 1 cup sliced English cucumber
- 1 cup thinly sliced red onions

Prep

1. Preheat the oven to 350 degrees. Combine the rosemary, thyme, chives, sea salt, and black pepper. Brush the top and sides of each salmon fillet with ½ tablespoon per salmon fillet of Dijon mustard, then season with the herb mixture. Spray a baking dish with cooking spray or cover with parchment paper.

Cook

2. Heat a skillet over medium-high heat and spray with cooking spray. Sear the salmon top-side down for 1 minute; gently flip the fillets and cook for another minute. Remove the salmon from the pan; sauté the mushrooms for 2 minutes. You may need to spray pan with more cooking spray prior to sautéing mushrooms.

3. Transfer the mushrooms to the prepared baking dish and put the salmon on top of the mushrooms. Bake for 12 minutes, or until the salmon reaches an internal temperature of 145 degrees.

Serve

4. To assemble, combine the kale and broccoli slaw in a large bowl. Top with diced cucumber, red onions, roasted mushrooms, and salmon.

Note:
This salad pairs well with the Red Pepper Dressing or Spicy Balsamic Vinaigrette. (see page 111 & 115)

Asian Chopped Salad
with Salmon

Ingredients

Salmon:

- 1 tablespoon olive oil
- 1 teaspoon onion powder
- 1 teaspoon ground garlic
- ½ teaspoon dried paprika
- ½ teaspoon Chili powder
- ¼ teaspoon ground cayenne pepper
- 1 teaspoon sea salt
- Cooking spray
- 4 (6 ounces each) salmon fillets

Salad Base:

- 7 cups spring mix
- 1 cup thinly sliced red cabbage
- 1 cup thinly sliced green onions
- 1 cup grated carrots
- 1 cup thinly sliced celery
- 1 cup chopped peanuts
- 1 cup diced red bell peppers
- Chopped cilantro (for garnish)

Prep

1. Preheat the oven to 400 degrees. Prepare the seasoning mixture by combining the olive oil, onion powder, garlic, paprika, chili powder, cayenne pepper, and sea salt. Set aside. Spray a sheet pan with cooking spray or line with parchment paper; put the salmon on top. Season the salmon by brushing on the prepared seasoning mixture.

Cook

2. Bake for 15 to 20 minutes, or until the salmon reaches an internal temperature of 145 degrees.

Serve

3. To assemble the salad, toss the spring mix and cabbage in a large bowl; top with arranged rows of the prepared green onions, carrots, celery, peanuts, and red peppers. Top with salmon, and garnish with cilantro.

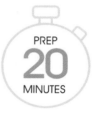

PREP
20
MINUTES

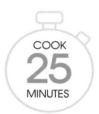

COOK
25
MINUTES

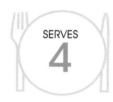

SERVES
4

Note:

This salad pairs well with the Cilantro Lime Dressing or Garlic Lime Dressing.
(see page 113)

e2mfitness.com

Jerk Shrimp
Salad

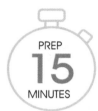

PREP
15
MINUTES

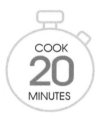

COOK
20
MINUTES

SERVES
4

Ingredients

Shrimp:
- 2 pounds (31/35) shrimp, fresh or frozen, peeled and deveined
- 1 tablespoon olive oil
- 2 tablespoons Jerk Seasoning (see page 121)

Salad Base:
- 8 cups chopped spring mix
- 1 cup thinly sliced red onions
- 1 cup thinly sliced bell peppers
- 1 cup carrots
- 2 avocados, peeled and diced
- 1 cup diced cucumber

Prep

1. For the Jerk Seasoning, combine all the ingredients and mix well; store in an airtight container.
2. If the shrimp is frozen, thaw in a colander under running water.
3. Combine the shrimp and 2 tablespoons of the Jerk Seasoning; toss to coat evenly.

Cook

4. Heat the olive oil in a skillet over medium-high heat. Add the seasoned shrimp; sauté the shrimp in batches until the shrimp turn pink, 2 to 3 minutes on each side. The shrimp will look like the letter C when raw and the letter G when fully cooked. Note that it is best to cook the shrimp in batches.

Serve

5. To assemble the salad, put the spring mix in a large bowl; top with prepared red onions, bell peppers, shrimp, carrots, avocado, and cucumber.

Note:
This salad pairs well with the Cilantro Lime Dressing. (see page 113)

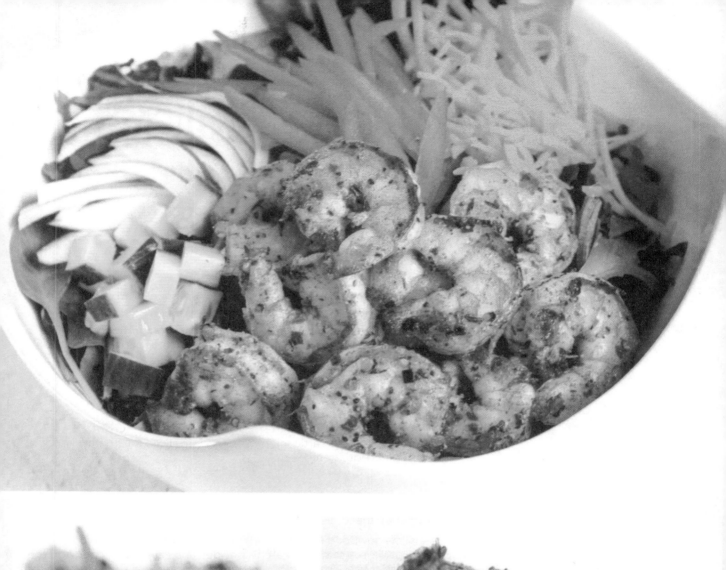

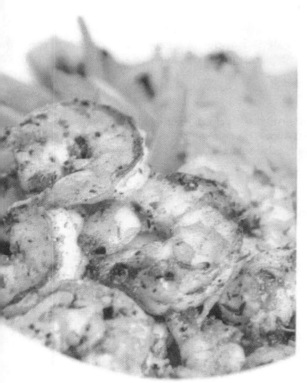

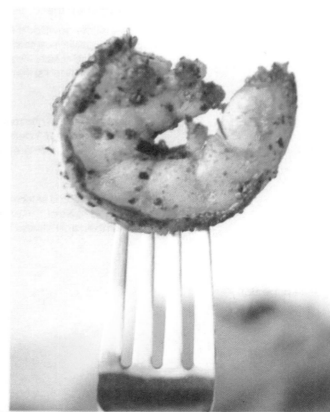

Greek Kale Salad
with Chicken

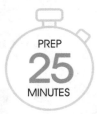

PREP
25
MINUTES

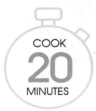

COOK
20
MINUTES

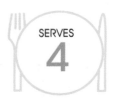

SERVES
4

Ingredients

Tempeh:
- 2 pounds chicken breast
- 1 tablespoon olive oil
- 1 teaspoon onion powder
- 1 teaspoon ground garlic
- 1 teaspoon sea salt
- ½ teaspoon dried paprika
- ½ teaspoon mild chili powder
- ¼ teaspoon ground cayenne pepper

Salad Base:
- 8 cups baby kale
- 1 cup thinly sliced red onions
- 1 cup chopped canned artichoke hearts, drained, quartered
- 1 cup grated carrots
- 1 cup diced cucumber
- ¼ cup sliced Kalamata olives

Prep

1. Preheat the oven to 400 degrees, and line a sheet pan with parchment paper.

2. In a shallow bowl, or baking dish, whisk together the olive oil, onion powder, garlic, sea salt, paprika, chili powder, and cayenne pepper. Add the chicken and toss to coat evenly. Arrange the chicken in a single layer on the parchment-lined sheet pan.

Cook

3. Bake for 10 to 15 minutes, or until the chicken reaches an internal temperature of 165 degrees. Allow the chicken to rest for 10 minutes, then dice the chicken to prepare for the salad.

Serve

4. To assemble the salad, put the baby kale into a large bowl; top with arranged rows of the prepared red onions, artichoke hearts, chicken, carrots, cucumber, and olives.

Note:
This salad pairs well with the Cilantro Lime Dressing.
(see page 113)

Chicken and Kale
Salad

Ingredients

Chicken:

- Cooking spray
- 2 pounds chicken breast
- 1 tablespoon olive oil
- 1 teaspoon onion powder
- 1 teaspoon ground garlic
- 1 tablespoon sea salt
- ½ teaspoon dried paprika
- ½ teaspoon chili powder
- ¼ teaspoon ground cayenne pepper

Salad Base:

- 8 cups baby kale
- 1 cup thinly sliced red onions
- 1 cup thinly sliced bell peppers
- 1 cup grated carrots
- 2 avocados, peeled and diced
- 1 cup diced cucumber

Prep

1. Preheat the oven to 350 degrees. Prepare a glass baking dish by spraying with cooking oil. Combine the chicken breast with the olive oil, onion powder, garlic, sea salt, paprika, chili powder, and cayenne pepper; mix well to coat the chicken evenly.

Cook

2. In a skillet over medium-high heat, spray with cooking oil. Add the chicken and cook for 3 to 4 minutes per side. Transfer the chicken to the prepared baking pan; finish cooking it in the oven for 10-15 minutes, or until the chicken reaches an internal temperature of 165 degrees. Allow the chicken to cool, then dice the chicken to prepare for the salad.

Serve

3. To assemble the salad, put the baby kale greens into a large bowl; top with arranged rows of thinly sliced red onions, bell peppers, chicken, carrots, avocado, and cucumber.

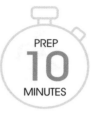

PREP
10
MINUTES

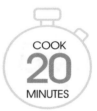

COOK
20
MINUTES

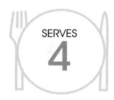

SERVES
4

Note:

This salad pairs well with the classic Italian Vinaigrette or Lemon Vinaigrette. (see page 110 & 111)

e2mfitness.com

Chopped Autumn Salad
with Turkey

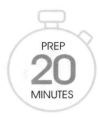

PREP
20
MINUTES

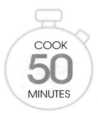

COOK
50
MINUTES

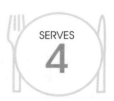

SERVES
4

Ingredients

Turkey:
- Cooking spray
- 2 pounds turkey tenderloin
- 1 teaspoon kosher salt
- ½ teaspoon fresh sage
- ½ teaspoon fresh thyme
- ½ teaspoon dried rosemary
- ¼ teaspoon black pepper

Salad:
- 4 cups spinach
- 4 cups shredded cabbage
- 1 cup thinly sliced red onions
- 1 cup shredded carrots
- 1 cup diced cucumber
- 1 cup diced celery
- 1 cup chopped pecans

Prep

1. Preheat the oven to 375 degrees. Spray a baking pan with cooking spray. Arrange the turkey tenderloins in the pan, and spray the turkey with cooking oil. In a small bowl, combine the kosher salt, sage, thyme, rosemary, and black pepper. Mix well, then rub all over the tenderloins.

2. Combine the spinach, cabbage, red onions, carrots, cucumber, and celery. Toss to combine.

Cook

3. Bake for 30 to 40 minutes, or until the seasoned tenderloins reach an internal temperature of 165 degrees. Allow the turkey to cool for 10 minutes, then slice.

Serve

4. To assemble the salad, plate the salad mix and top with turkey and pecans.

Note:
This salad pairs well with the Lemon Vinaigrette or Garlic Lime Dressing.
(see page 111 & 113)

e2mfitness.com

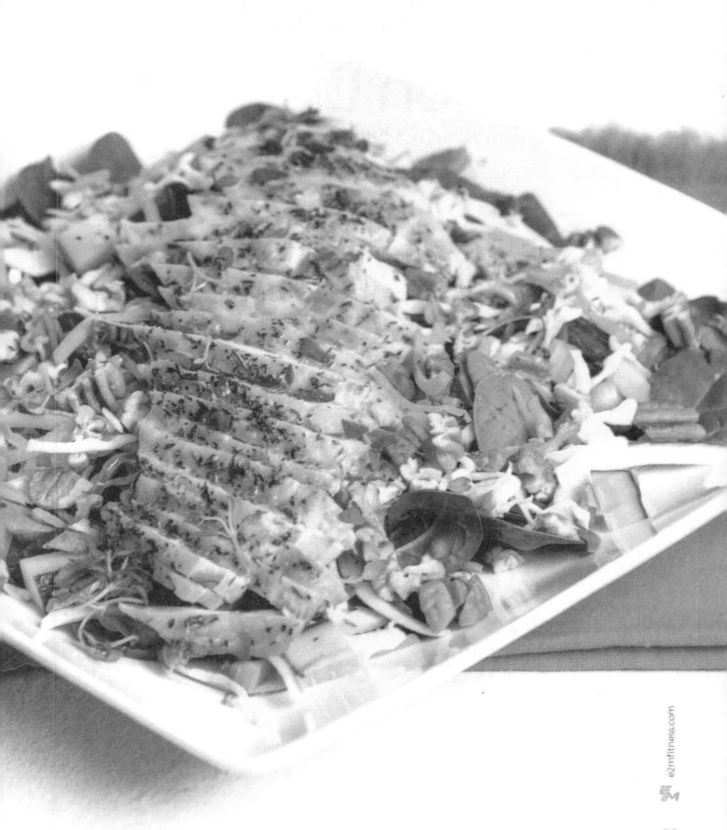

Salmon Blueberry
Avocado Salad

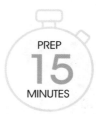

PREP
15
MINUTES

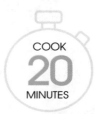

COOK
20
MINUTES

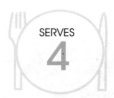

SERVES
4

Ingredients

Salmon:
- 4 (6 ounces each) salmon fillets
- 1 teaspoon onion powder
- 1 teaspoon ground garlic
- 1 teaspoon sea salt
- ½ teaspoon dried paprika
- ½ teaspoon mild chili powder
- ¼ teaspoon ground cayenne pepper
- Cooking spray

Salad Base:
- 8 cups baby spinach
- 1 cup diced red onions
- 1 cup grated carrots
- 1 cup thinly sliced cucumber
- 2 avocados, peeled and diced
- 1 cup fresh blueberries
- Crushed red pepper (for garnish)

Prep

1. Preheat the oven to 400 degrees. In a small bowl, combine the onion powder, garlic, sea salt, paprika, chili powder, and cayenne pepper. Spray cooking oil on a sheet pan, then put the salmon on top. Spray the salmon with a small amount of cooking spray; season the salmon with the spice blend.

Cook

2. Bake for 15 to 20 minutes, or until the salmon reaches an internal temperature of 145 degrees.

Serve

3. To assemble the salad, put the baby spinach in a large bowl; top with diced red onions, carrots, cucumber, avocado, and blueberries; top with salmon and garnish with crushed red pepper.

Note:
This salad pairs well with the Lemon Vinaigrette or Cilantro Lime Dressing.
(see page 111 & 113)

e2mfitness.com

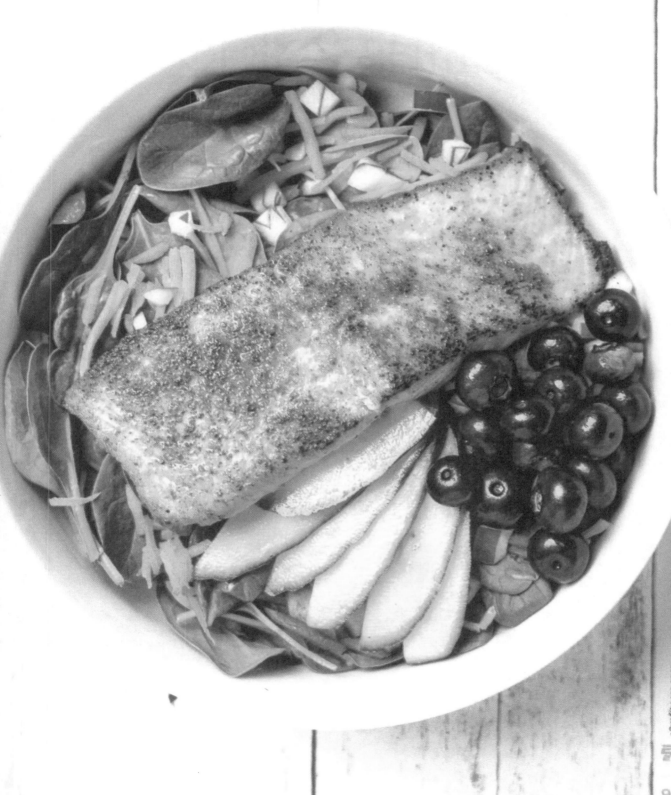

Citrus Salad
with Pecan-Crusted Salmon

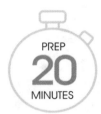

PREP
20
MINUTES

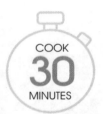

COOK
30
MINUTES

SERVES
4

Ingredients

Salmon:
- 4 (6 ounces each) fresh salmon fillets
- ½ teaspoon sea salt
- ½ teaspoon black pepper
- Cooking spray
- 2 tablespoons Dijon mustard
- ½ cup chopped pecans
- 1 tablespoon dried thyme
- 2 tablespoons chopped fresh parsley
- 2 tablespoons orange zest (use an orange from salad base)

Salad Base:
- 4 cups baby kale
- 4 cups shaved brussels sprouts
- 4 oranges
- 1 red onion, thinly sliced

Prep

1. Preheat the oven to 350 degrees. Line an oven-safe dish with parchment paper or spray with cooking oil.
2. Season the salmon with sea salt and black pepper.

Cook

3. Heat a pan over medium-high heat; spray with cooking oil. Sear the salmon top side down for 1 minute; gently flip the fillets and cook for another minute. Remove the salmon and let rest to cool slightly. Spread 1½ teaspoons of the Dijon mustard over each fillet.
4. Combine the pecans, thyme, parsley, and orange zest on a plate; roll each salmon fillet in the herb-nut mixture. Put the fillets on the prepared pan; bake for 12 to 15 minutes, or until the salmon reaches an internal temperature of 145 degrees.
5. Toss the baby kale and shaved brussels sprouts in a large bowl. Cut off the top and bottom of each orange, and peel down the sides to remove the white pith from the oranges; cut the oranges crosswise into segments.

Serve

6. To assemble the salad, divide the kale and brussels sprouts mixture bet plates; add a portion of the thinly sliced red onions and sliced oranges to each serving; top with the salmon.

Note:
This salad pairs well with the Spicy Balsamic Dressing.
(see page 115)

e2mfitness.com

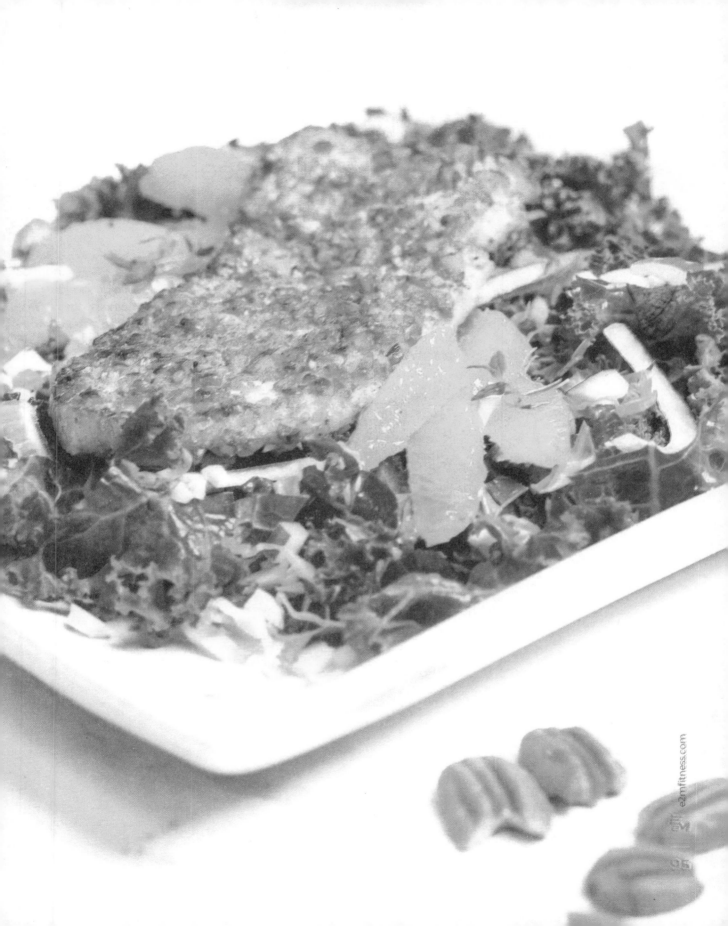

Thai Salad
with Ginger Ground Beef

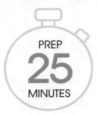

PREP
25
MINUTES

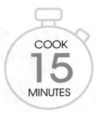

COOK
15
MINUTES

SERVES
4

Ingredients

Beef:

- Cooking spray
- 2 pounds lean ground beef (90% lean)
- 2 green onions, chopped
- 1 teaspoon ground garlic
- 2 teaspoons sea salt
- 1 teaspoon sesame oil
- ½ teaspoon ground ginger
- ½ teaspoon crushed red pepper
- 2 tablespoons water

Salad Base:

- 7 cups spring mix
- 1 cup thinly sliced red cabbage
- 1 cup thinly sliced celery
- 1 cup grated carrots
- 1 cup thinly sliced cucumber
- 1 cup chopped peanuts
- 1 cup diced red bell peppers
- Chopped cilantro (for garnish)

Cook

1. Heat a skillet over medium heat and spray with cooking oil. Add the ground beef, stirring to break up the meat. Add the chopped green onions, garlic, sea salt, sesame oil, ginger, crushed red pepper, and water; mix well. Continue cooking until the beef is cooked through. The ground beef is done when it reaches an internal temperature of 160 degrees, 10 to 12 minutes.

Serve

2. To assemble the salad, toss the spring mix and cabbage in a large bowl; top with arranged rows of the prepared celery, carrots, cucumber, peanuts, and red pepper. Add the ground beef and garnish with cilantro.

Note:
This salad pairs well with the Thai Peanut Dressing.
(see page 117)

e2mfitness.com

Mandarin Chicken
Salad

Ingredients

Chicken:
- 2 pounds chicken breast
- 1 tablespoon Lemon Pepper Seasoning (see page 120)
- 1 tablespoon olive oil
- 1 teaspoon dried basil
- 1 teaspoon dried oregano
- 1 teaspoon sea salt
- ½ teaspoon dried thyme
- Cooking spray

Salad Base:
- 8 cups spinach
- ¼ cup thinly sliced green onions
- 4 mandarins, peeled and separated
- 1 cup diced cucumber
- ½ cup slivered almonds
- Black and white sesame seeds (for garnish)

Prep

1. Preheat the oven to 400 degrees. Combine the chicken, Lemon Pepper Seasoning, olive oil, basil, oregano, sea salt, and thyme; mix well to coat the chicken evenly. Refrigerate for 20 minutes to marinate. Spray cooking oil on a sheet pan or line with parchment paper, and put the seasoned chicken on the pan.

Cook

2. Bake for 10 to 15 minutes, or until the chicken reaches an internal temperature of 165 degrees. Allow the chicken to rest for 10 minutes, then dice the chicken to prepare for the salad.

Serve

3. To assemble the salad, put the spinach in a large bowl; add the thinly sliced green onions, diced cucumber, mandarin orange segments, and slivered almonds; top with chicken and then sesame seeds for garnish.

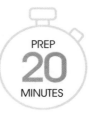

PREP
20
MINUTES

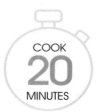

COOK
20
MINUTES

SERVES
4

Note:
This salad pairs well with the Red Pepper Dressing or Cilantro Lime Dressing.
(see page 111 & 113)

e2mfitness.com

Buffalo-"Ranch"
Chicken Salad

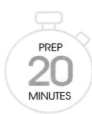

PREP
20
MINUTES

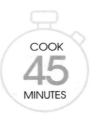

COOK
45
MINUTES

SERVES
4

Ingredients

Chicken:
- 2 tablespoons olive or avocado oil
- 2 pounds chicken breast or tenders

Salad base:
- 8 cups shredded cabbage
- 1 cup sliced celery
- 1½ cups shredded carrots
- 2 avocados, peeled and diced
- ¼ cup chopped cilantro
- 1 tablespoon olive oil
- 1 tablespoon lemon juice
- 1 tablespoon dill

Seasonings:
- 2 tablespoons "Ranch" Seasoning (see page 121)
- Buffalo Seasoning (see page 127)

Prep

1. For the salad base, combine the cabbage, celery, and carrots in a large bowl.

2. Prepare the "Ranch" Seasoning in a small bowl by combining the garlic, thyme, parsley, dill, cilantro, sea salt, and black pepper; add 2 tablespoons of the blend to the salad base with 1 tablespoon olive oil and 1 tablespoon lemon juice and toss to mix. Store the extra seasoning blend in an airtight container.

3. For the Buffalo Seasoning, combine the chili powder, paprika, onion powder, garlic, sea salt, black pepper, and optional cayenne pepper; mix well.

Cook

4. To cook the chicken, pour oil into a deep sided pot; add the Buffalo Seasoning over medium heat to "bloom" the spices and develop flavor. Allow to heat until you start to smell the spices. Add 3 to 4 cups of water; bring the water to a boil and add the chicken. Make sure the chicken is covered with the liquid. Boil for 20 minutes; remove the chicken and allow to slightly cool.

5. Shred the chicken with a hand mixer or with two forks, pulling apart. Add a tablespoon of the cooking liquid to the shredded chicken.

Serve

6. To assemble the salad, first divide the cabbage mixture between 4 plates; add the shredded chicken and diced avocado. Top with fresh cilantro.

Note:
This salad pairs well with the Vegan "Ranch" Dressing. (see page 116)

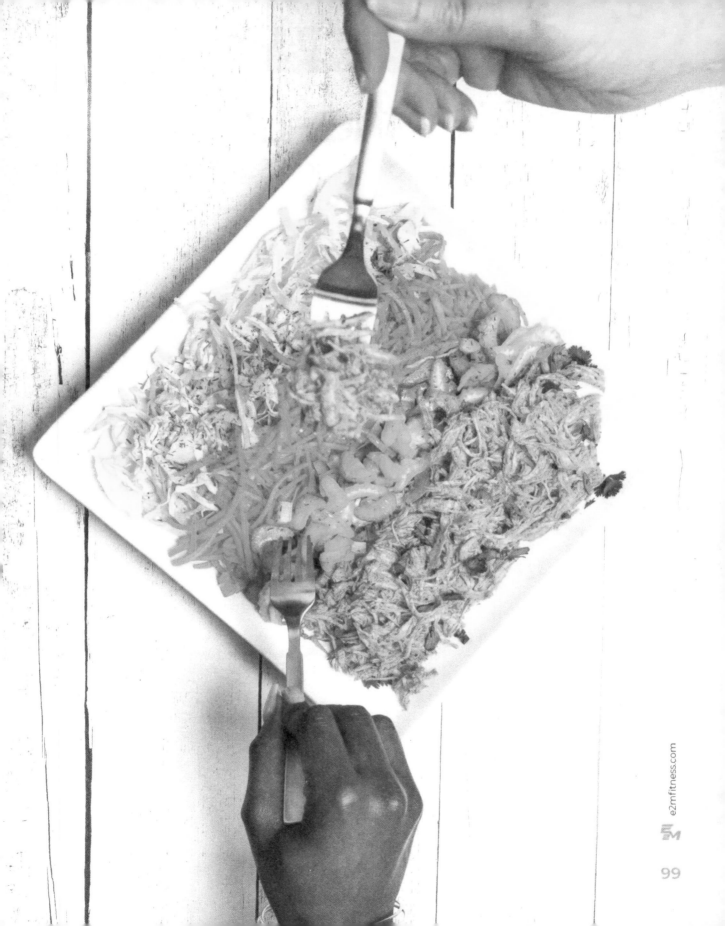

Cilantro-Lime
Roasted Salmon Salad

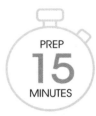

PREP
15
MINUTES

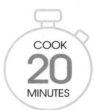

COOK
20
MINUTES

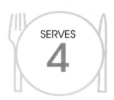

SERVES
4

Ingredients

Roasted Salmon Salad:

- 4 (6 ounces each) salmon fillets
- Cooking spray
- ¼ teaspoon sea salt
- ⅛ teaspoon black pepper
- 6 cups chopped spinach
- 2 cups arugula
- 1 cucumber, diced
- 2 avocados, peeled and diced
- 1 lime, zested and juiced
- 2 tablespoons chopped cilantro
- 2 tablespoons Chili-Lime Seasoning (see page 120)

Chili-Lime Seasoning:

- ½ teaspoon dried smoked paprika
- ½ teaspoon ground garlic
- ½ teaspoon black pepper
- ½ teaspoon dried oregano
- ¼ teaspoon ground cayenne pepper
- 1 teaspoon sea salt
- 1 teaspoon chili powder
- 1 teaspoon olive oil
- Zest from 1 lime

Prep

1. Preheat the oven to 400 degrees. Spray sheet pan with cooking oil or line it with parchment paper. Spray the salmon with the cooking spray; season with sea salt, black pepper, and Chili-Lime Seasoning. Then put the fillets on the prepared pan.

Cook

2. Roast for 15 to 20 minutes. Broil for 2 to 3 minutes. The salmon should reach an internal temperature of 145 degrees.

Serve

3. To assemble the salad, combine the spinach, arugula, cucumber, avocado, and salmon; divide between the plates. Top with a squeeze of lime juice and zest with fresh cilantro.

Note:

This salad pairs well with Red Pepper Dressing or Cilantro Lime Dressing.
(see page 111 & 113)

e2mfitness.com

"Ranch" Shrimp
Salad

Ingredients

Shrimp:

- 2 pounds (31/35) shrimp, fresh or frozen, peeled and deveined
- ½ red onion, finely diced
- 1 cucumber, sliced
- 1 tablespoon rice vinegar
- 1 tablespoon Everything Seasoning (see page 125)
- Cooking spray
- "Ranch" Seasoning (recipe below)

Salad Base:

- 8 cups spring mix
- 2 avocados, peeled and diced
- 1 cup mandarin orange segments
- 1 lemon, zested and juiced

"Ranch" Seasoning:

- 1 teaspoon ground garlic
- 1 teaspoon dried parsley
- 2 teaspoons dried dill
- ¼ teaspoon dried thyme
- 1 lemon, zested and juiced
- ½ teaspoon sea salt
- ⅛ teaspoon black pepper

Prep

1. If the shrimp is frozen, thaw in a colander under running water.

2. Prepare the "ranch" seasoning in a large bowl by combining the garlic, parsley, dill, thyme, lime zest, lime juice, sea salt, and black pepper. Add the shrimp; toss to coat evenly.

3. In a separate bowl, combine the prepared red onion and cucumber with the rice vinegar and Everything seasoning; refrigerate until ready to serve.

Cook

4. Heat a pan over medium heat and spray with cooking oil. Add the seasoned shrimp; sauté the shrimp in batches until the shrimp turn pink, 2 to 3 minutes on each side. The shrimp will look like the letter C when raw and the letter G when fully cooked. Note that it is best to cook the shrimp in batches.

Serve

5. To assemble the salad, combine the cucumber and onion mixture with the shrimp, spring mix, and diced avocado. Top with mandarin orange segments, lemon zest, and lemon juice.

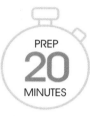

**PREP
20
MINUTES**

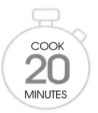

**COOK
20
MINUTES**

**SERVES
4**

Note:
This salad pairs well with scratch-made Vegan "Ranch" Dressing.
(see page 116)

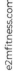

Shrimp and Peach
Summer Salad

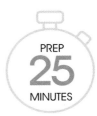

PREP
25
MINUTES

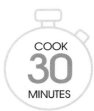

COOK
30
MINUTES

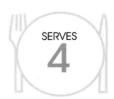

SERVES
4

Note:
Deglazing simply means to add liquid to a hot pan and use a wooden spoon to remove any cooked-on food. This creates a flavorful "sauce" you can cook vegetables in for added flavor.

Note:
This salad pairs well with Chipotle Chimichurri Vinaigrette (see page 110)

Ingredients

Shrimp:

- 2 pounds (31/35) shrimp, fresh or frozen, peeled and deveined
- 2 lemons, zested and juiced
- ½ tablespoon crushed red pepper
- ½ teaspoon fresh garlic, minced
- 1 tablespoon olive oil
- 1 teaspoon sea salt
- ½ teaspoon black pepper

Salad Base:

- 3 English cucumbers, halved and sliced
- 8 cups chopped spinach
- 2 cups diced celery
- ¼ cup chopped fresh basil
- ¼ teaspoon sesame seeds
- ¼ teaspoon crushed red pepper (optional)
- Cooking spray
- 2 peaches, pitted and quartered
- 2 avocados, peeled and diced

Prep

1. If the shrimp is frozen, thaw in a colander under running water.

2. In a large bowl, whisk together the lemon juice and zest, crushed red pepper, garlic, olive oil, sea salt, and black pepper. Add the shrimp and refrigerate for 30 minutes.

3. Combine the spinach, cucumber, celery, and basil with the sesame seeds and optional crushed red pepper. Toss to mix well.

Cook

4. Heat a pan over medium heat. Spray the pan with cooking oil; sauté the peaches for 2 to 3 minutes and remove from the pan. Add a squeeze of lemon juice from 1/2 lemon to deglaze the pan.

5. Add the seasoned shrimp; sauté the shrimp in batches until the shrimp turn pink, 2 to 3 minutes on each side. The shrimp will look like the letter C when raw and the letter G when fully cooked. Note that it is best to cook the shrimp in batches.

Serve

6. To assemble the salad, divide the cucumber salad between plates; top each plate with a portion of the shrimp, sautéed peaches, and diced avocado.

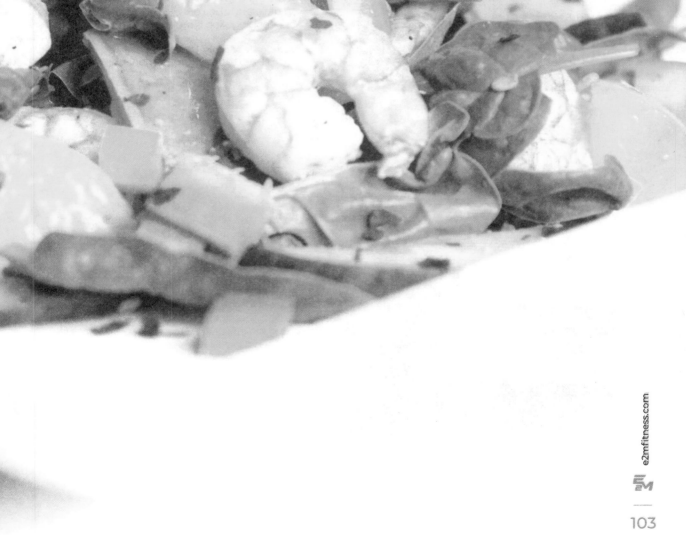

⧉ Success Stories

Scott W., Fredonia, NY

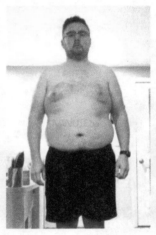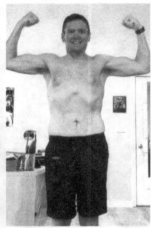

Rounds	Age	Weight Loss
3	35	90

As a pastor, I want to set an example for others. E2M fitness has taught me self-discipline on a whole new level. I was overweight my whole life. I was the kid who would go out of his way to skip gym class. I would drown my sorrows in cookies and every junk food I could get my hands on. Now I finally see myself as an athlete. My kids are making healthier choices. Our congregation is making healthier choices.

Non-Scale Victory (NSV)!
I can fit into seats on amusement park rides with my kids!

Sara H., Lexington, SC

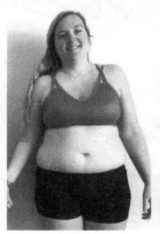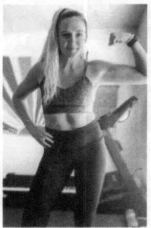

Rounds	Age	Weight Loss
7	31	50

I was tired of being tired. I was tired of not wanting to take part in fun things with my children because it was too "stressful." Stressful was my excuse for being uncomfortable in my own skin, always being too hot, always hating how my clothes fit, always having a headache from soda addiction and, of course, not wanting to be in pictures.

How has E2M fitness changed your life?
I'm a better wife and mother because of the E2M program. I have the energy to play with my children and complete daily tasks. I have a newfound confidence that makes me excited about social events.

Mediterranean
Cobb Salad

Ingredients

- 12 eggs
- 4 cups baby kale
- 4 cups packaged broccoli slaw
- 1⅓ cups chopped red bell peppers
- 1⅓ cups chopped bella mushrooms
- 1⅓ cups chopped canned artichoke hearts, drained

Prep

1. To make hard-boiled eggs, arrange the eggs in a single layer at the bottom of a saucepan; add enough water to completely cover the eggs.

Cook

2. Bring the water to a rolling boil; turn off the heat, cover, and let sit. Depending on how you prefer your hard-boiled eggs, remove the eggs from the water after 8 to 10 minutes (for softer yolks) or 10 to 12 minutes (for firmer yolks). Submerge the eggs in cold water to stop the cooking process, and peel.

Serve

3. To assemble the salad, combine the kale and broccoli slaw; divide between 4 plates. Top each serving with 3 sliced hard-boiled eggs and a portion of the prepared red peppers, mushrooms, and artichokes.

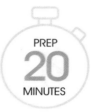

PREP
20
MINUTES

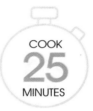

COOK
25
MINUTES

SERVES
4

Note:
This salad pairs well with the Avocado Lime Dressing or Vegan "Ranch" Dressing.
(see page 115 & 116)

e2mfitness.com

Sonoma Chicken
Salad

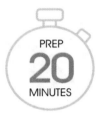

PREP
20
MINUTES

COOK
25
MINUTES

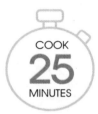

SERVES
4

Ingredients

Chicken:

- 2 pounds chicken tenders
- 1 tablespoon dried basil
- 1 tablespoon dried rosemary
- 1 tablespoon olive oil
- Cooking spray
- ½ tablespoon sea salt
- ½ tablespoon black pepper
- 1 tablespoon fresh thyme

Salad Base:

- 4 cups chopped romaine
- 4 cups shredded cabbage or slaw mixture
- 2 cups chopped apples
- ½ cup finely chopped celery
- ½ cup chopped red onions
- ½ lemon, juiced
- ½ cup chopped pecans

Prep

1. With a paper towel, pat dry the chicken; slice the chicken into strips if using the breast. Put into a bowl. Add 1 tablespoon olive oil, basil, rosemary, thyme, salt, and pepper on the chicken. Toss to combine.

Cook

2. Heat a skillet over medium-high heat and spray with cooking spray; sauté the chicken for 5 to 8 minutes on each side until the chicken reaches an internal temperature of 165 degrees. Set aside and allow to cool.

Serve

3. To assemble the salad, put the romaine and shredded cabbage into a large bowl, then add the chicken and the prepared apples, celery, red onions, and lemon juice. Toss to combine; top with pecans.

Note:
This salad pairs well with the Chipotle Chimichurri Vinaigrette or Red Pepper Dressing. (see page 110 & 111)

e2mfitness.com

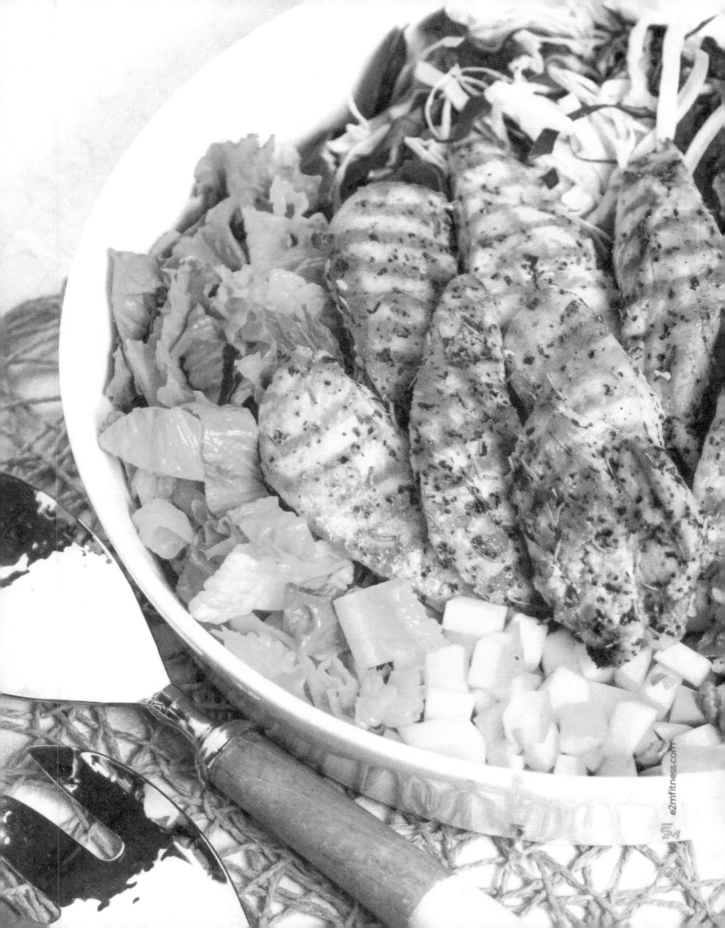

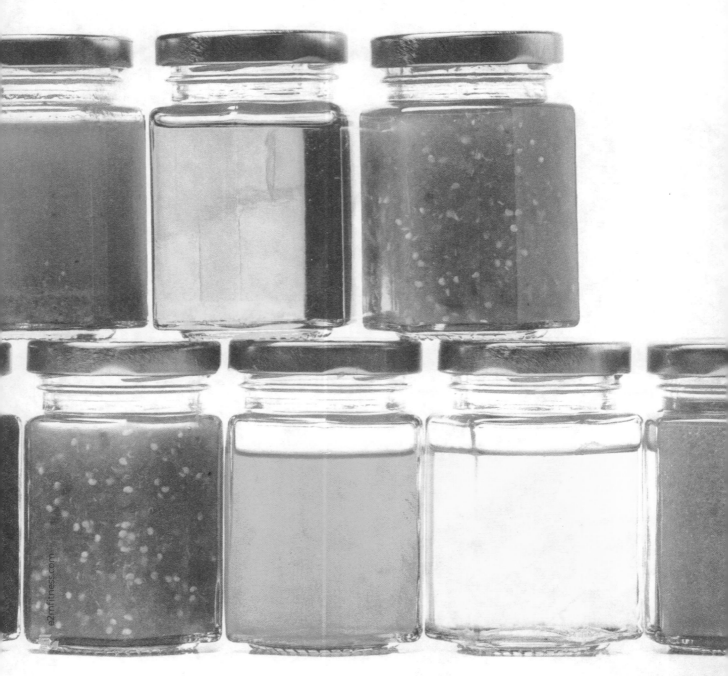

Dressings made from scratch are versatile and simple to make at home. Any of these dressing recipes can also be used as marinades for your proteins. These ingredients are used in many other recipes, so go ahead and buy in bulk to stock your pantry!

Another major benefit of homemade dressings is that they are free of preservatives, added sugars, and artificial flavorings. The more you know, the more you grow!

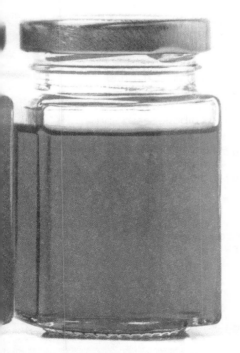

Dressings

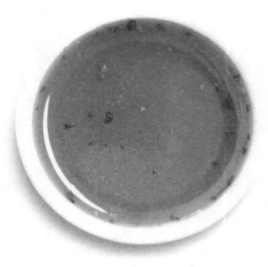

Italian Vinaigrette

½ cup extra-virgin olive oil
2 tablespoons red wine vinegar
1 teaspoon Dijon mustard
¼ teaspoon dried parsley
¼ teaspoon dried oregano
2 fresh garlic cloves, minced
⅛ teaspoon crushed red pepper
¼ teaspoon sea salt
⅛ teaspoon black pepper

Combine all ingredients in a mason jar, secure the lid, and shake. Store in an airtight container in the refrigerator for up to three days.

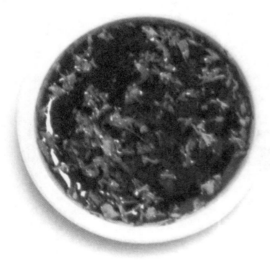

Chipotle Chimichurri Vinaigrette

½ cup extra virgin olive oil
2 tablespoons fresh lime juice
2 tablespoons red wine vinegar
2 fresh garlic cloves, minced
¼ cup fresh flat-leaf parsley, chopped
½ cup fresh cilantro, chopped
¼ teaspoon sea salt
¼ teaspoon ground chipotle seasoning

Combine all ingredients in a blender. Blend until smooth. Store in an airtight container in the refrigerator for up to three days.

Chef Note: pairs deliciously with chicken or beef.

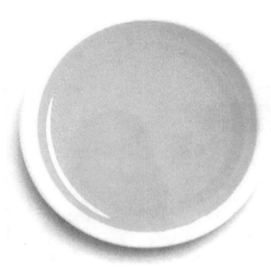

Lemon Vinaigrette

½ cup extra-virgin olive oil
3 tablespoons fresh lemon juice
1 teaspoon Dijon mustard
2 fresh garlic cloves, minced
¼ teaspoon sea salt
⅛ teaspoon black pepper

Combine all ingredients in a mason jar, secure the lid, and shake. Store in an airtight container in the refrigerator for up to three days.

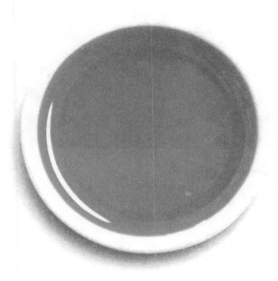

Red Pepper Dressing

½ cup extra-virgin olive oil
½ cup canned roasted red peppers, drained
¼ cup lemon juice
1 tablespoon Dijon mustard
1 fresh garlic clove, minced
½ teaspoon sea salt
¼ teaspoon black pepper

Combine all ingredients in a blender. Blend until smooth. Store in an airtight container in the refrigerator for up to three days.

⧉ Success Stories

Dawain A., Fayetteville, NC

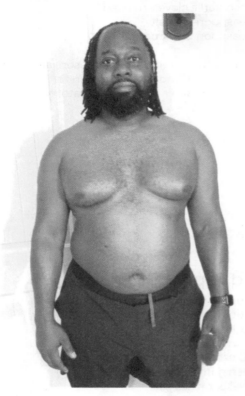 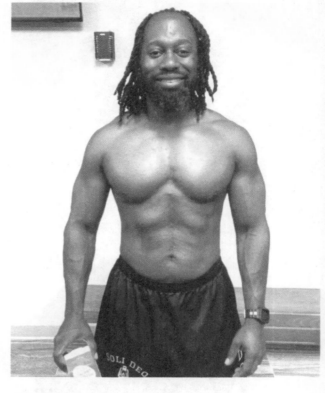

Rounds	Age	Weight Loss
7	40	65

E2M fitness has reminded me that I "get" to workout and that moving my body is a privilege. I was on the road to high blood pressure and diabetes. Now I've gained my health back.

What does the E2M community mean to you?
The E2M community is like family to me. We cheer each other on, we encourage and motivate one another, and we challenge each other. It's a beautiful thing to see people from all walks of life come together, forgetting the things that separate us while pursuing a common goal of fitness.

Non-Scale Victory (NSV)!
I went from not being able to walk a mile to running a 5K.

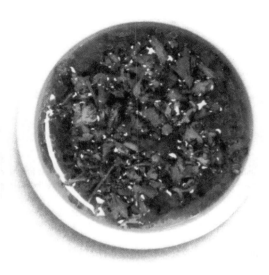

Cilantro Lime Dressing

½ cup extra-virgin olive oil
2 tablespoons fresh lime juice
1 tablespoon apple cider vinegar
1 teaspoon fresh garlic, minced
¼ cup fresh cilantro, chopped
¼ teaspoon sea salt
⅛ teaspoon black pepper

Combine all ingredients in a blender. Blend until smooth. Store in an airtight container in the refrigerator for up to three days.

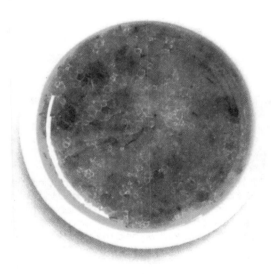

Garlic Lime Dressing

½ cup extra-virgin olive oil
1 tablespoon rice vinegar
1 teaspoon ground garlic
1 teaspoon fresh parsley
1 teaspoon dried dill
2 limes, zest and juice
¼ teaspoon sea salt
⅛ teaspoon black pepper

Combine all ingredients in a mason jar (only the zest and juice from the lime are used), secure the lid, and shake. Store in an airtight container in the refrigerator for up to three days.

Success Stories

Jessica M., Wilmington, NC

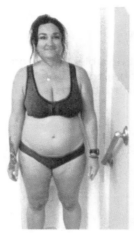 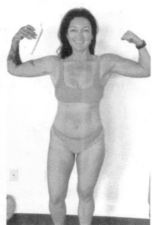

Rounds	Age	Weight Loss
7	31	46

I initially wanted to lose twenty pounds. I lost that and then some and I've gained so much more from joining this E2M program than I ever expected. It's fantastic to look and feel stronger. I just FEEL good every day and that is something I haven't ever felt! I am so grateful for the coaches, chefs, and everyone involved with this wonderful program. It truly has changed my life for the better.

Non-Scale Victory (NSV)!
My cheekbones are back, and I can hold a plank for three minutes!

Bradley B., Jamestown, NY

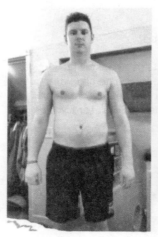 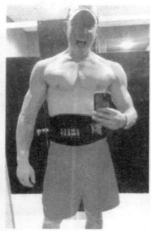

Rounds	Age	Weight Loss
2	34	20

E2M fitness has changed my life by reminding me that every day is an opportunity to excel and to continually invest in my overall well-being. I've almost completely given up alcohol and started focusing on filling my body with foods that will help me feel my best.

Non-Scale Victory (NSV)!
Being able to train for over four hours in preparation for the Maryland Full Ironman.

What is your favorite type of workout?
Strength training through HIIT circuits and weightlifting.

Spicy Balsamic Vinaigrette

3 tablespoons balsamic vinegar
½ cup extra-virgin olive oil
1 tablespoon Dijon mustard
1 teaspoon ground garlic
⅛ teaspoon chipotle seasoning
¼ teaspoon sea salt
⅛ teaspoon black pepper

Combine all ingredients in a mason jar, secure the lid, and shake. Store in an airtight container in the refrigerator for up to three days.

Avocado Lime Dressing

½ cup extra-virgin olive oil
1 avocado, peeled and diced
3 tablespoons lime juice
1 tablespoon apple cider vinegar
¼ cup cilantro, chopped
1 teaspoon Dijon mustard
¼ teaspoon sea salt
⅛ teaspoon black pepper

Combine all ingredients in a blender. Blend until smooth. Store in an airtight container in the refrigerator for up to three days.

Creamy Tahini Dressing

¼ cup water
¼ cup tahini
3 tablespoons lemon juice
1 fresh garlic clove, minced
½ teaspoon Dijon mustard
¼ teaspoon sea salt
⅛ teaspoon black pepper

Combine all ingredients in a blender. Blend until smooth. Store in an airtight container in the refrigerator for up to three days.

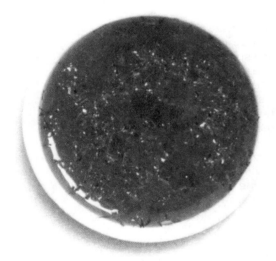

Vegan "Ranch" Dressing

½ cup extra-virgin olive oil
¼ cup rice wine vinegar
1 teaspoon ground garlic
1 tablespoon fresh parsley
1 teaspoon dried dill
¼ teaspoon dried thyme
1 lime, zest and juice
1 tablespoon chopped fresh cilantro
¼ teaspoon sea salt
⅛ teaspoon black pepper

Combine all ingredients in a blender (only the zest and juice from the lime are used). Blend until smooth. Store in an airtight container in the refrigerator for up to three days.

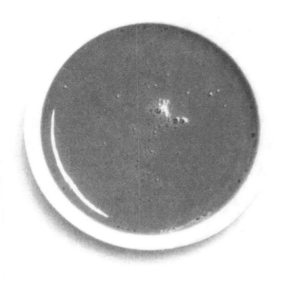

Thai Peanut Dressing

¼ cup peanut butter
3 tablespoons lime juice
1 tablespoon soy sauce
2 teaspoons fresh grated ginger
½ teaspoon chili paste
1 garlic clove, minced
¼ teaspoon sea salt
⅛ teaspoon black pepper

Combine all ingredients in a blender.
Blend until smooth. Add water as
needed to thin the sauce to your desired
consistency. Season with sea salt and black
pepper. Store in an airtight container in
the refrigerator for up to three days.

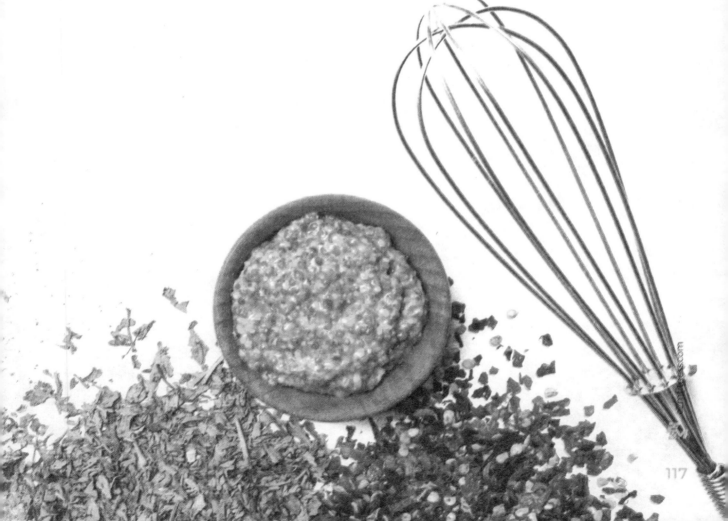

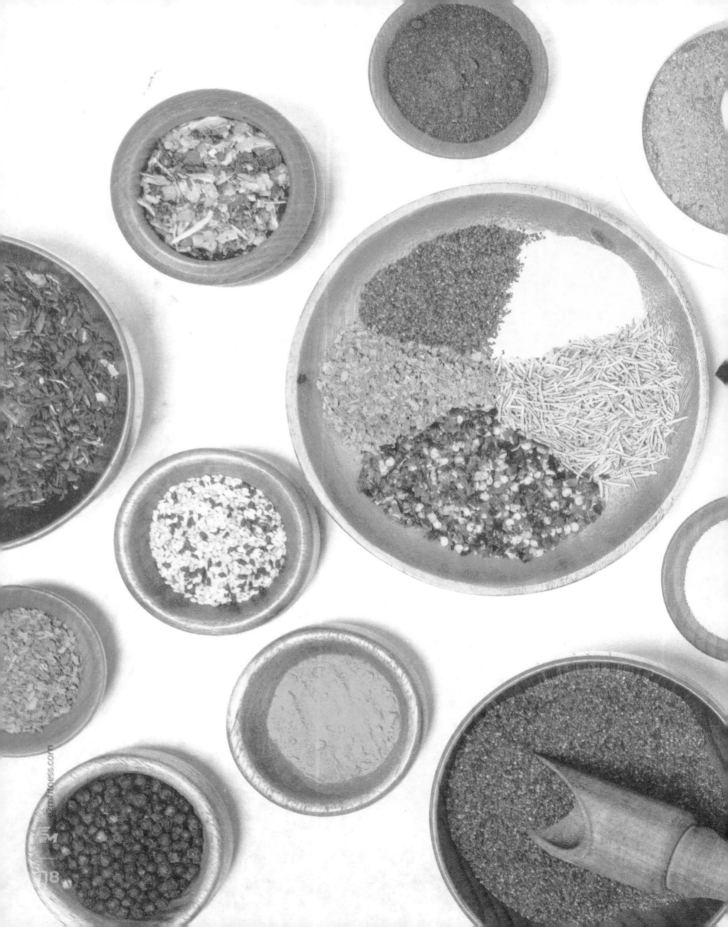

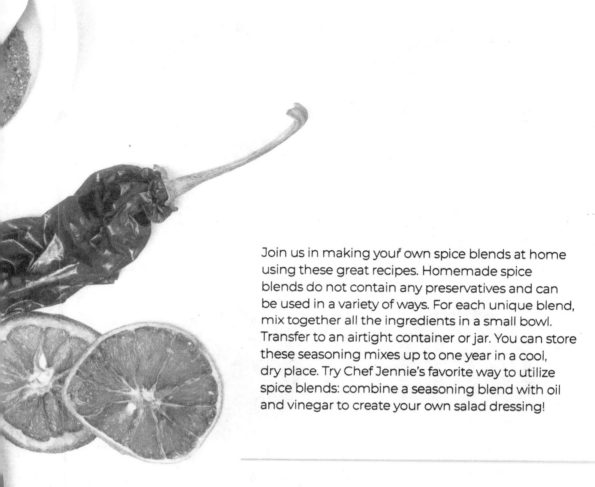

Join us in making your own spice blends at home using these great recipes. Homemade spice blends do not contain any preservatives and can be used in a variety of ways. For each unique blend, mix together all the ingredients in a small bowl. Transfer to an airtight container or jar. You can store these seasoning mixes up to one year in a cool, dry place. Try Chef Jennie's favorite way to utilize spice blends: combine a seasoning blend with oil and vinegar to create your own salad dressing!

Spice Blends

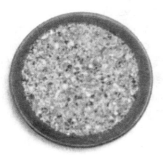

Mediterranean Blend

1 teaspoon ground garlic
½ teaspoon sea salt
½ teaspoon dried rosemary
½ teaspoon dried oregano
½ teaspoon black pepper
½ teaspoon lemon zest

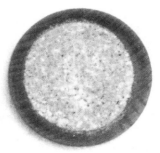

Ginger Garlic Blend

1 tablespoon ground ginger
1½ teaspoons ground garlic
1 teaspoon black pepper
¼ teaspoon sea salt

Lemon Pepper Seasoning

1 tablespoon lemon zest
1½ teaspoons ground
   rainbow peppercorn
½ teaspoon onion powder
½ teaspoon ground garlic

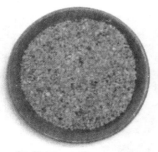

Chili-Lime Seasoning

½ teaspoon dried
   smoked paprika
½ teaspoon ground garlic
½ teaspoon black pepper
½ teaspoon dried oregano
¼ teaspoon ground
   cayenne pepper
1 teaspoon sea salt
1 teaspoon chili powder
Zest from 1 lime

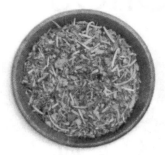

Herbs de Provence Seasoning

1 tablespoon dried thyme
1 tablespoon dried basil
1½ teaspoons dried oregano
1 teaspoon dried rosemary
½ teaspoon dried tarragon

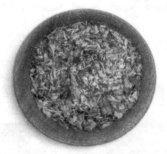

"Ranch" Seasoning

1½ tablespoons ground garlic
1 tablespoon dried thyme
1 tablespoon dried parsley
1 tablespoon dried dill
1 tablespoon dried cilantro
⅛ teaspoon sea salt
⅛ teaspoon black pepper

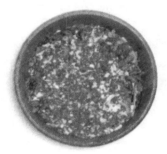

Jerk Seasoning

1 tablespoon ground garlic
2 teaspoons ground cayenne pepper
2 teaspoons onion powder
2 teaspoons dried thyme
2 teaspoons dried parsley
2 teaspoons sea salt
1 teaspoon dried paprika
1 teaspoon ground allspice
½ teaspoon black pepper
½ teaspoon crushed red pepper
½ teaspoon ground nutmeg
¼ teaspoon ground cinnamon

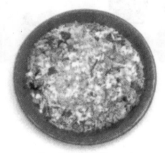

Peri Peri Blend

2 teaspoons dried paprika
2 teaspoons ground cayenne pepper
2 teaspoons ground garlic
2 teaspoons dried oregano
1 teaspoon sea salt
1 teaspoon crushed red pepper
½ teaspoon ground cinnamon
½ teaspoon ground cardamom
½ teaspoon ground ginger

⧖ Success Stories

Justin B., Salisbury, NC

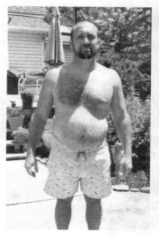 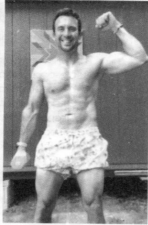

Rounds	Age	Weight Loss
6	40	40

I was a college athlete who let life get in the way of my health and fitness. I was always trying to outwork a poor diet. I was tired of being tired and the E2M fitness program changed my life!

What did you want to change about your lifestyle?
I wanted to feel good and look good!

What does the E2M community mean to you?
I LOVE to read about people's individual stories and see how the E2M fitness program has paved the way for them to take back their life.

Berri H., Simpscnville, SC

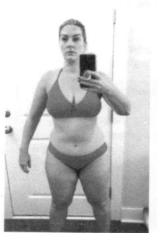 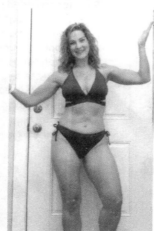

Rounds	Age	Weight Loss
5	45	40

I came to the E2M program seeking mental clarity and a better way to manage stress. I was looking for that connection between exercising and the brain. It didn't even occur to me that I could stick with it to lose weight. I am an overthinker and I need explicit instructions when taking on something new. E2M fitness provided that strict (effective) direction for me: eat this, not that.

Non-Scale Victory (NSV)!
I sleep better, my skin is better, my clothing size stays consistent, I have more energy, I'm stronger, and my confidence is through the roof!

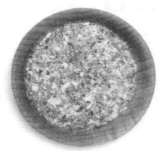

Lemon Basil Seasoning

1 tablespoon lemon zest
1½ teaspoons dried basil
1 teaspoon sea salt
1 teaspoon ground garlic
½ teaspoon dried thyme
½ teaspoon black pepper

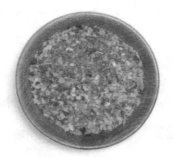

Cajun Blend

2½ teaspoons dried paprika
2 teaspoons ground garlic
1½ teaspoons sea salt
1¼ teaspoons dried oregano
1¼ teaspoons dried thyme
1 teaspoon onion powder
1 teaspoon ground
    cayenne pepper
1 teaspoon black pepper
½ teaspoon crushed red pepper

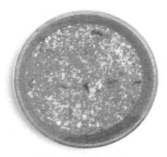

Spicy BBQ Rub

1 teaspoon chili powder
1 teaspoon ground garlic
¼ teaspoon ground cumin
¼ teaspoon ground mustard
¼ teaspoon sea salt
⅛ teaspoon black pepper
⅛ teaspoon ground
    cayenne pepper
⅛ teaspoon crushed red pepper
⅛ teaspoon chipotle seasoning

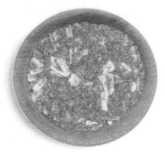

Smoked Chili Seasoning

2 tablespoons chili powder
1 tablespoon dried
    smoked paprika
1 tablespoon ground cumin
1 tablespoon dried oregano
1 tablespoon ground garlic
1 tablespoon onion powder

Ⴔ Success Stories

Shuntoya L., Mebane, NC

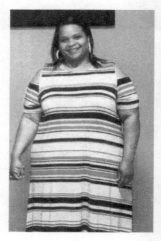 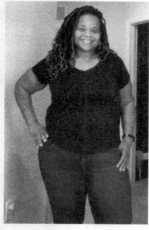

Rounds	Age	Weight Loss
3	44	77

I've been dealing with diabetes and prediabetes for many years and my weight loss with the E2M program has totally removed me from being in the diabetic range. This has changed my life in so many ways. I anticipate having a much longer life now and I look forward to seeing my son grow up.

What is your biggest E2M accomplishment?
My biggest accomplishment has been to consistently work out six days per week. This is the first time in my life that I've been able to accomplish this level of consistency.

Nicole C., Mount Holly, NC

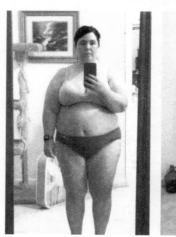 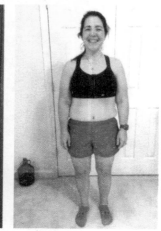

Rounds	Age	Weight Loss
8	49	73

I was put on a diet when I was ten months old and I have struggled with my weight ever since. At six years old, I had a nutritionist, but I couldn't understand what she was saying. When I was older, I'd work out, but I had no idea of the nutrition aspect, so I'd eventually give up. I just needed someone to tell me what to eat and what to do and that I could do it!

Non-Scale Victory (NSV)!
I can do hard things every day!

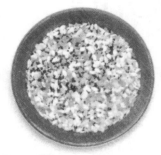

Everything Seasoning

2 tablespoons ground garlic
2 tablespoons onion powder
½ teaspoon poppy seeds
½ teaspoon sesame seeds
½ teaspoon black pepper
¼ teaspoon sea salt

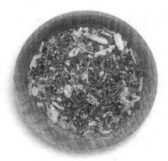

Southwestern Seasoning

2 tablespoons chili powder
1 tablespoon ground cumin
1 tablespoon dried oregano
1 tablespoon ground garlic
1 tablespoon onion powder

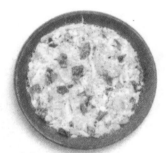

Asian Spice Blend

1½ tablespoons ground garlic
1½ teaspoons sea salt
1½ teaspoons ground ginger
1½ teaspoons crushed red pepper
1½ teaspoons black pepper
1½ teaspoons onion powder

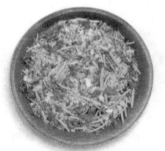

Lemon Herb Spice Blend

1 teaspoon dried paprika
1 teaspoon dried rosemary
½ teaspoon sea salt
½ teaspoon black pepper
¼ teaspoon ground garlic
¼ teaspoon dried parsley
¼ teaspoon ground mustard
¼ teaspoon onion powder
Zest from 1 lemon

⧱ Success Stories

LC C., Marietta, GA

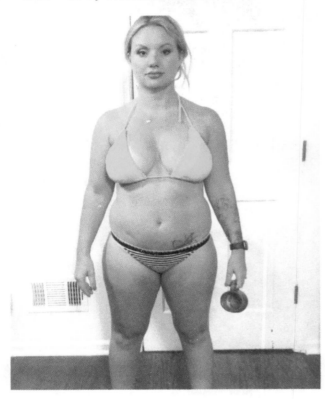
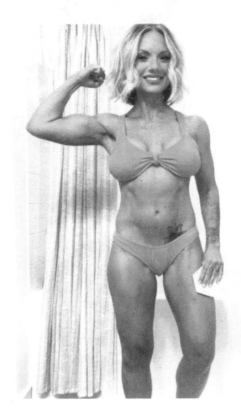

Rounds	Age	Weight Loss
6	**37**	**55**

When joining E2M fitness, I wanted to change my relationship with food and alcohol. I used drinking to numb anxiety and stress. I used food as a coping mechanism and to celebrate. Ten years ago, I was hit by a drunk driver while walking on a sidewalk and was told I may never walk again. I was tired of knee injections and anti-inflammatories. I wanted to get up and celebrate my body, not pick it apart in a mirror every day.

Non-Scale Victory (NSV)!
My orthopedic took me off all pain medicines for my knees and I ran a 10K!

Additional
Spice Blends

Buffalo Seasoning

1 teaspoon chili powder
1 teaspoon dried paprika
½ teaspoon onion powder
½ teaspoon ground garlic
½ teaspoon sea salt
¼ teaspoon black pepper
¼ teaspoon ground
    cayenne pepper

Greek Seasoning

2 tablespoons dried oregano
1 tablespoon dried dill
1 tablespoon ground garlic
1 tablespoon onion powder
½ teaspoon sea salt
¼ teaspoon black pepper

Adobo Seasoning

1 tablespoon sea salt
1 tablespoon dried
    Spanish paprika
2 teaspoons black pepper
2 teaspoons ground garlic
1 teaspoon onion powder
1 teaspoon dried oregano
1 teaspoon chili powder
1 teaspoon ground cumin

Veggie Seasoning

3 tablespoons onion powder
1 tablespoon ground garlic
1 tablespoon sea salt
1 teaspoon black pepper
1 teaspoon dried thyme
1 teaspoon dried paprika
½ teaspoon dried parsley

Curry Powder

4 teaspoons ground coriander
2 teaspoons ground turmeric
2 teaspoons ground mustard
2 teaspoons chili powder
1 teaspoon sea salt
1 teaspoon ground
    cayenne pepper
1 teaspoon ground cumin
½ teaspoon ground cardamom

Garlic and Herb
Seasoning

¼ cup kosher salt
1 tablespoon ground garlic
1 tablespoon lemon zest
2 teaspoons dried rosemary
1½ teaspoons dried thyme
1½ teaspoons dried oregano
¼ teaspoon dried paprika
¼ teaspoon crushed
    red pepper

Seafood Spice Blend

½ tablespoon salt
1 tablespoon celery seed
1½ teaspoons sweet paprika
1 teaspoon ground dry mustard
1 teaspoon ground ginger
5 bay leaves, ground
½ teaspoon smoked paprika
½ teaspoon black pepper
¼ teaspoon crushed red pepper
⅛ teaspoon ground nutmeg
⅛ teaspoon ground cardamom
⅛ teaspoon ground allspice
⅛ teaspoon ground cinnamon
1 pinch of ground cloves

Thai Spice Blend

2 teaspoons dried paprika
1 teaspoon ground turmeric
1 teaspoon black pepper
1 teaspoon ground coriander
1 teaspoon ground fenugreek
1 teaspoon sea salt
½ teaspoon dry mustard
½ teaspoon ground cumin
½ teaspoon ground ginger
⅛ teaspoon ground
    cayenne pepper

e2mfitness.com

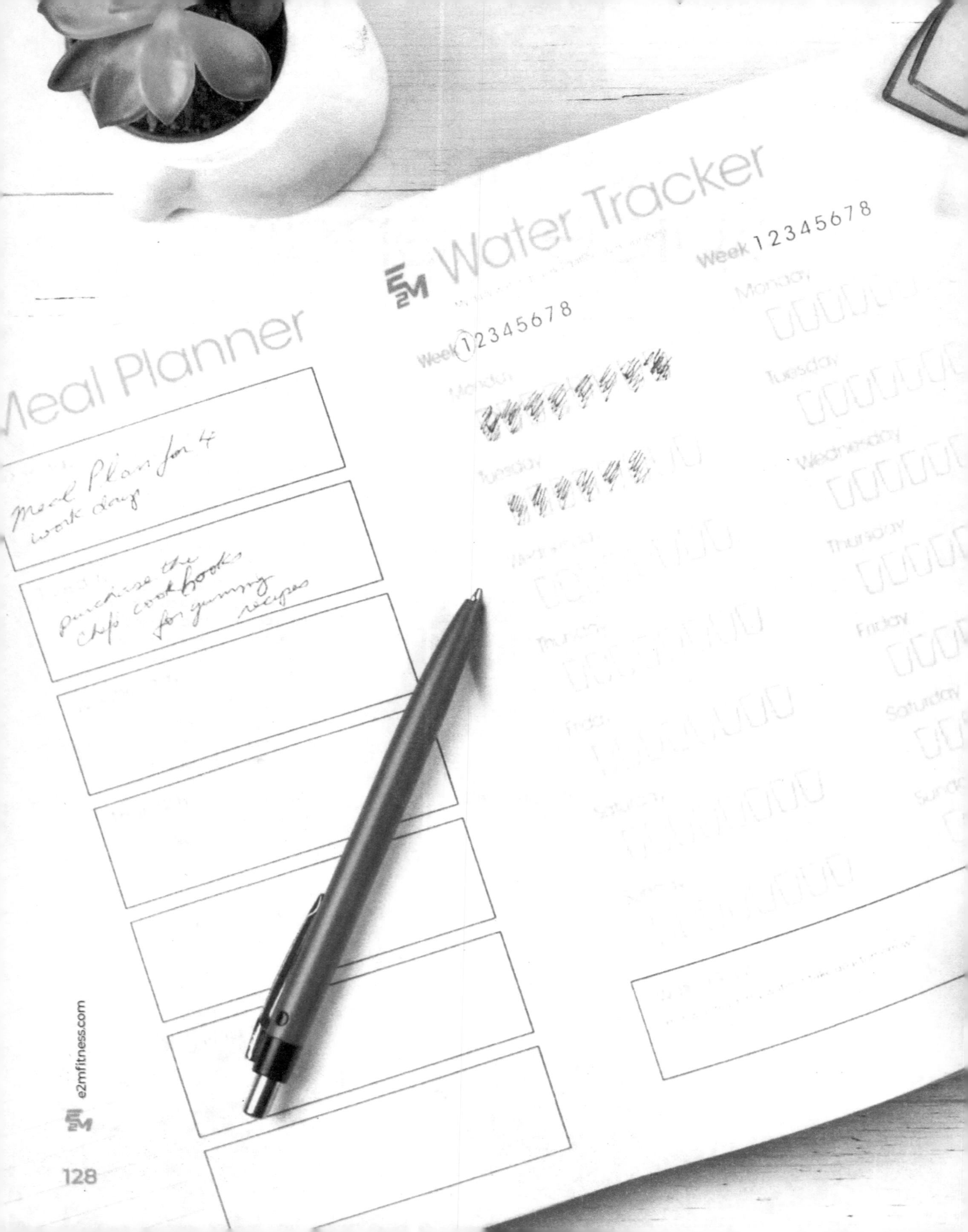

Meal Planner

Meal Plan for 4
work days

purchase the
E2 cookbooks
for yummy
recipes

Water Tracker

Monday

Tuesday

Thursday

Friday

Saturday

Monday

Tuesday

Wednesday

Thursday

Friday

Saturday

Sunday

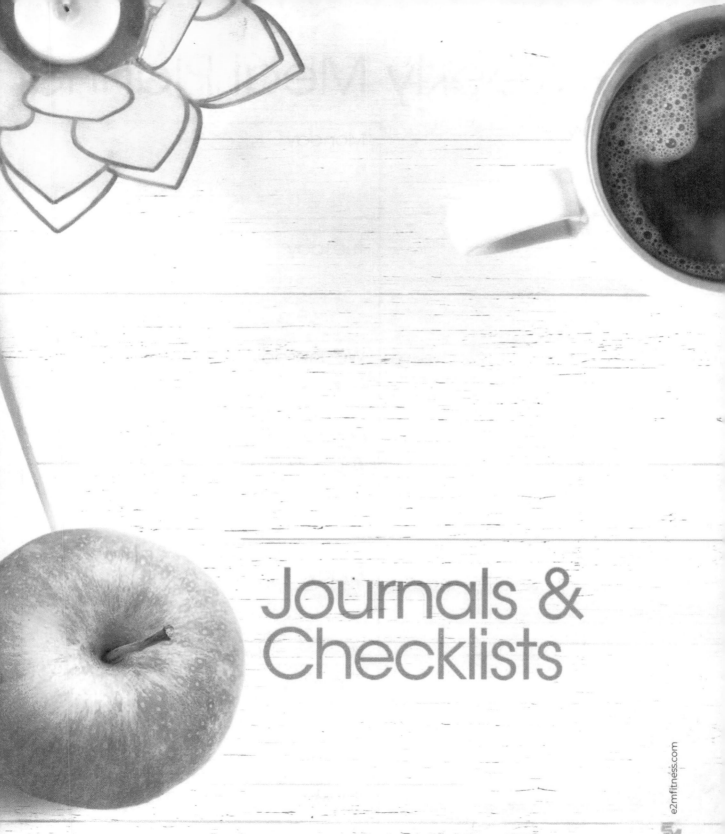

Journals & Checklists

Weekly Meal Planner

Grocery List

Veggies

_____
_____
_____
_____
_____
_____

Protein

_____
_____
_____
_____
_____

Other

_____
_____
_____
_____

Monday

Tuesday

Wednesday

Thursday

Friday

Saturday

Sunday

Water Tracker

My daily water goal is 1 gallon (128 ounces).

Week 1 2 3 4 5 6 7 8

Monday

Tuesday

Wednesday

Thursday

Friday

Saturday

Sunday

Week 1 2 3 4 5 6 7 8

Monday

Tuesday

Wednesday

Thursday

Friday

Saturday

Sunday

Water Goals:

How will I reach my water intake goal tomorrow?

Each glass represents 16 oz.

Weekly Exercise

Monday	Tuesday

Wednesday	Thursday

Friday	Saturday

Sunday	Non-Scale Victory for the week:
	YAY ME!

Me vs. Me! Trust the Process!

Monthly Habits

Check or color in the square for the new healthy habits you completed.

	Meal Prep	Meal 1	Meal 2	Meal 3	Mindfulness	Workout 1	Workout 2	Jeff's Live	Water Goal	Celebration Meal	Journal
Day 1											
Day 2											
Day 3											
Day 4											
Day 5											
Day 6											
Day 7											
Day 8											
Day 9											
Day 10											
Day 11											
Day 12											
Day 13											
Day 14											
Day 15											
Day 16											
Day 17											
Day 18											
Day 19											
Day 20											
Day 21											
Day 22											
Day 23											
Day 24											
Day 25											
Day 26											
Day 27											
Day 28											
Day 29											
Day 30											
Day 31											

⧟ Weekly Meal Planner

Grocery List

Veggies

_____

_____

_____

_____

_____

_____

_____

Protein

_____

_____

_____

_____

_____

_____

_____

Other

_____

_____

_____

_____

Monday

Tuesday

Wednesday

Thursday

Friday

Saturday

Sunday

Water Tracker

My daily water goal is 1 gallon (128 ounces).

Week 1 2 3 4 5 6 7 8

Monday
⊔ ⊔ ⊔ ⊔ ⊔ ⊔ ⊔ ⊔

Tuesday
⊔ ⊔ ⊔ ⊔ ⊔ ⊔ ⊔ ⊔

Wednesday
⊔ ⊔ ⊔ ⊔ ⊔ ⊔ ⊔ ⊔

Thursday
⊔ ⊔ ⊔ ⊔ ⊔ ⊔ ⊔ ⊔

Friday
⊔ ⊔ ⊔ ⊔ ⊔ ⊔ ⊔ ⊔

Saturday
⊔ ⊔ ⊔ ⊔ ⊔ ⊔ ⊔ ⊔

Sunday
⊔ ⊔ ⊔ ⊔ ⊔ ⊔ ⊔ ⊔

Week 1 2 3 4 5 6 7 8

Monday
⊔ ⊔ ⊔ ⊔ ⊔ ⊔ ⊔ ⊔

Tuesday
⊔ ⊔ ⊔ ⊔ ⊔ ⊔ ⊔ ⊔

Wednesday
⊔ ⊔ ⊔ ⊔ ⊔ ⊔ ⊔ ⊔

Thursday
⊔ ⊔ ⊔ ⊔ ⊔ ⊔ ⊔ ⊔

Friday
⊔ ⊔ ⊔ ⊔ ⊔ ⊔ ⊔ ⊔

Saturday
⊔ ⊔ ⊔ ⊔ ⊔ ⊔ ⊔ ⊔

Sunday
⊔ ⊔ ⊔ ⊔ ⊔ ⊔ ⊔ ⊔

Water Goals:

How will I reach my water intake goal tomorrow?

e2mfitness.com

⊔ Each glass represents 16 oz.

⚡ Weekly Exercise

Monday	Tuesday
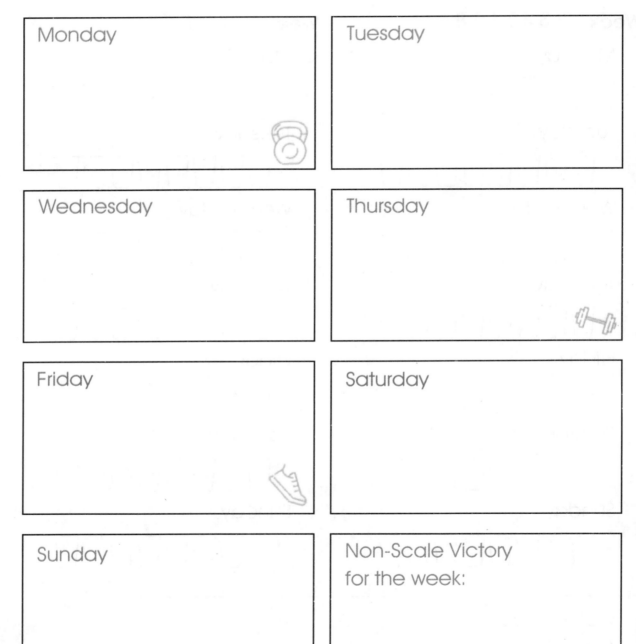	

Wednesday	Thursday

Friday	Saturday

Sunday	Non-Scale Victory for the week:
	YAY ME!

Me vs. Me! Trust the Process!

Monthly Habits

Check or color in the square for the new healthy habits you completed.

	Meal Prep	Meal 1	Meal 2	Meal 3	Mindfulness	Workout 1	Workout 2	Jeff's Live	Water Goal	Celebration Meal	Journal
Day 1											
Day 2											
Day 3											
Day 4											
Day 5											
Day 6											
Day 7											
Day 8											
Day 9											
Day 10											
Day 11											
Day 12											
Day 13											
Day 14											
Day 15											
Day 16											
Day 17											
Day 18											
Day 19											
Day 20											
Day 21											
Day 22											
Day 23											
Day 24											
Day 25											
Day 26											
Day 27											
Day 28											
Day 29											
Day 30											
Day 31											

Weekly Meal Planner

Grocery List

Veggies

_____

_____

_____

_____

_____

_____

Protein

_____

_____

_____

_____

_____

_____

Other

_____

_____

_____

_____

Monday

Tuesday

Wednesday

Thursday

Friday

Saturday

Sunday

Water Tracker

My daily water goal is 1 gallon (128 ounces).

Week 1 2 3 4 5 6 7 8

Monday

Tuesday

Wednesday

Thursday

Friday

Saturday

Sunday

Week 1 2 3 4 5 6 7 8

Monday

Tuesday

Wednesday

Thursday

Friday

Saturday

Sunday

Water Goals:

How will I reach my water intake goal tomorrow?

Each glass represents 16 oz.

⇉ Weekly Exercise

Monday	Tuesday
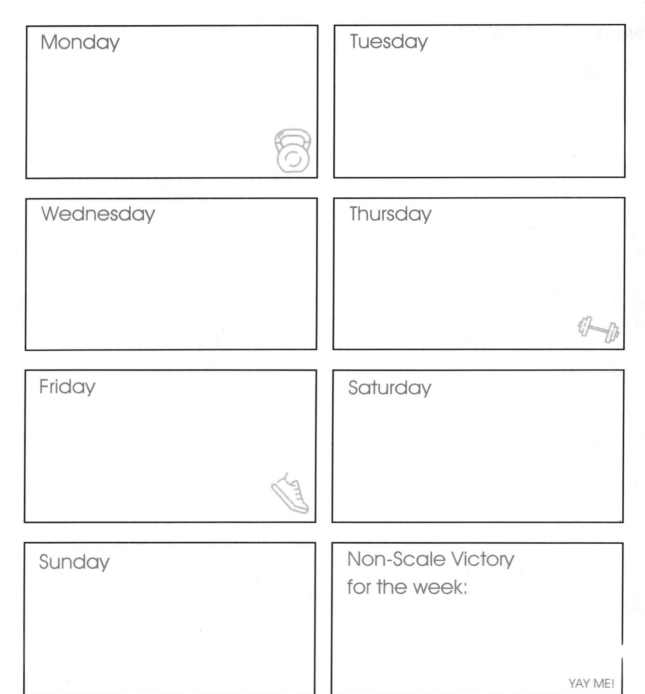	

Wednesday	Thursday

Friday	Saturday

Sunday	Non-Scale Victory for the week:
	YAY ME!

Me vs. Me! Trust the Process!

Monthly Habits

Check or color in the square for the new healthy habits you completed.

	Meal Prep	Meal 1	Meal 2	Meal 3	Mindfulness	Workout 1	Workout 2	Jeff's Live	Water Goal	Celebration Meal	Journal
Day 1											
Day 2											
Day 3											
Day 4											
Day 5											
Day 6											
Day 7											
Day 8											
Day 9											
Day 10											
Day 11											
Day 12											
Day 13											
Day 14											
Day 15											
Day 16											
Day 17											
Day 18											
Day 19											
Day 20											
Day 21											
Day 22											
Day 23											
Day 24											
Day 25											
Day 26											
Day 27											
Day 28											
Day 29											
Day 30											
Day 31											

Weekly Meal Planner

Grocery List

Veggies

_____

_____

_____

_____

_____

_____

Protein

_____

_____

_____

_____

_____

Other

_____

_____

_____

_____

_____

Monday

Tuesday

Wednesday

Thursday

Friday

Saturday

Sunday

Water Tracker

My daily water goal is 1 gallon (128 ounces).

Week 1 2 3 4 5 6 7 8

Monday

Tuesday

Wednesday

Thursday

Friday

Saturday

Sunday

Week 1 2 3 4 5 6 7 8

Monday

Tuesday

Wednesday

Thursday

Friday

Saturday

Sunday

Water Goals:

How will I reach my water intake goal tomorrow?

Each glass represents 16 oz.

Weekly Exercise

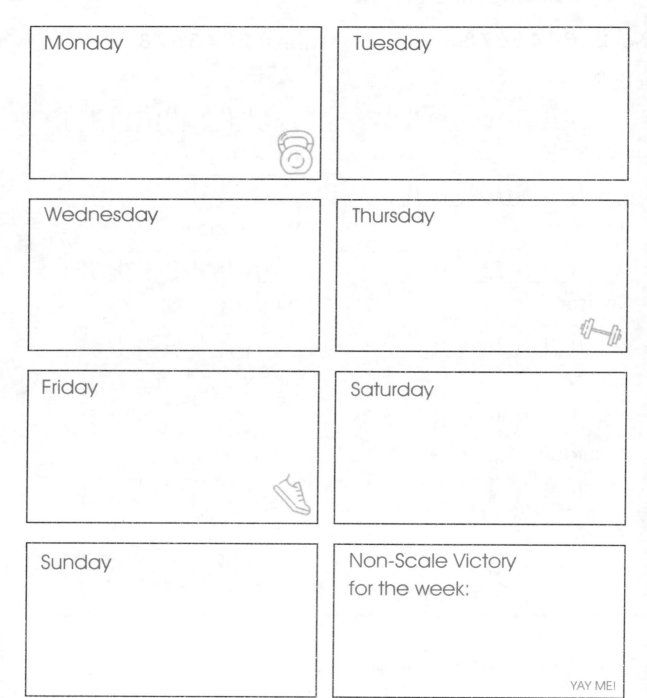

Monday

Tuesday

Wednesday

Thursday

Friday

Saturday

Sunday

Non-Scale Victory
for the week:

YAY ME!

Me vs. Me! Trust the Process!

e2mfitness.com

Monthly Habits

Check or color in the square for the new healthy habits you completed.

	Meal Prep	Meal 1	Meal 2	Meal 3	Mindfulness	Workout 1	Workout 2	Jeff's Live	Water Goal	Celebration Meal	Journal
Day 1											
Day 2											
Day 3											
Day 4											
Day 5											
Day 6											
Day 7											
Day 8											
Day 9											
Day 10											
Day 11											
Day 12											
Day 13											
Day 14											
Day 15											
Day 16											
Day 17											
Day 18											
Day 19											
Day 20											
Day 21											
Day 22											
Day 23											
Day 24											
Day 25											
Day 26											
Day 27											
Day 28											
Day 29											
Day 30											
Day 31											

e2mfitness.com